Binding Up
The
BROKENHEARTED

A HANDBOOK OF HOPE FOR THE CHRONICALLY* ILL & DISABLED

*Chronic: Marked by long duration or frequent recurrence, always present or encountered constantly: vexing, weakening, or troubling.

Webster's Seventh

Binding Up
The
BROKENHEARTED

A HANDBOOK OF HOPE FOR THE CHRONICALLY ILL & DISABLED

Cynthia L. Moench

COLLEGE PRESS PUBLISHING COMPANY
Joplin, Missouri

Library of Congress Catalog Card Number: 91-72136
International Standard Book Number: 0-89900-399-0

DEDICATION

For Jim: who not only said the words "For better, for worse . . . in sickness and in health," but *meant* them. Your tender care was at times all that kept me going. As Grandma Black would say, God broke the mold after He made you.

To Gaye: who cared enough to see that the time for grieving was over, and gently invited me to grow. Thank You.

And to all of those who stuck by me, suffered with me and prayed mightily for me. You know who you are.

AUTHOR'S NOTE

I am not going to debate the "issue" of healing here. If you are reading this and consider yourself chronically ill or disabled, then you more than likely have reached some understanding about God's divine healing or lack of it in your life. There are those who have built ministries and entire denominations around that one point – healing . . . and there are big-name preachers who claim to have been miraculously healed at some point in their lives. I will not dispute what these brothers and sisters in the Lord claim is *their experience*. We can never negate someone else's experience in total love.

But it is *their* experience, and as of yet, it has not been mine. My God is mighty, and he might choose tomorrow to heal me completely, and believe me, you'd not hear me complaining. The point is that He has not chosen to heal me yet, and I believe I'm being told, "Wait," or possibly even, "No."

God in His wisdom has one of these three answers for us at all times: "Yes," "No," or "Wait." But, of course, we all only want "Yes" answers.

C.M.

"The Lord is near to the brokenhearted and saves those who are crushed in spirit"
Psalm 34:18

"The Spirit of the Lord God is upon me, because the Lord has anointed me to bring good news to the afflicted; He has sent me to bind up the brokenhearted."
Isaiah 61:1

God doesn't give

explanations . . .

He gives promises

TABLE OF CONTENTS

DO I TRUST YOU, LORD?

by Twila Paris © 1984 by Singspiration Music
Used by permission of the
Benson Company, Inc., Nashville, Tennessee

Sometimes my little heart can't understand
What's in Your will, what's in Your plan,
So many times I'm tempted to ask You why.
But I can never forget it for long
Lord, what You do could not be wrong
So I believe You even when I must cry.

Do I trust You, Lord,
Does the river flow?
Do I trust You, Lord
Does the north wind blow?
You can see my heart,
You can read my mind
And You've got to know I would rather die
Than to lose my faith in the One I love
Do I trust You, Lord?

I know the answers, I've given them all
But suddenly now, I feel so small,
Shaken down to the cavity in my soul.
I know the doctrine and theology
But right now they don't mean much to me.
This time there's only one thing I've got to know.

(Cont'd)

Do I trust You, Lord
Does the robin sing–
Do I trust You, Lord
Does it rain in spring?
You can see my heart, You can read my mind
And You've got to know I would rather die
Than to lose my faith in the One I love
Do I trust You, Lord?

I will trust You, Lord
When I don't know why
I will trust You, Lord
Till the day I die
I will trust You, Lord
When I'm blind with pain
You were God before
And You'll never change.

I will trust You,
I will trust You,
I will trust You, Lord.

—Written for Melody Green after a plane
crash took the lives of her husband Keith,
(the founder of Last Days Ministries), and
their children.

1

THAT DREADED WORD, INCURABLE

The meaning of health: Health is defined by some as the absence of illness. As a psychological state, health is characterized by a feeling of well-being, vitality, and vigorous pursuit of life goals. Sickness is characterized by feelings of helplessness, dependency, continuous discomfort, and narrowing of attention.[1]

I picked up the phone one day to hear an unfamiliar voice at the other end. He told me that his name was Tim, he was 26 years old, and he had been given my name by a mutual friend. Although the call was coming from 2,000 miles away, I could tell that his voice was weak and he was near tears. "I know that you're ill, so I wanted to talk to you," he said. "I'm so scared and miserable. I just don't know what to do," he blurted out.

His tenderness and honesty touched me deeply as he went on to explain that he had just been diagnosed with Chronic Epstein-Barr Virus Syndrome (also known as Chronic Fatigue Syndrome). This young man was an elementary school teacher who loved his job and loved children. He also had an ill and elderly mother to care for. "I can't work. I can't function." Raw pain came searing through his voice. "Tell me, what am I going to do?"

I asked him if he had been able to get any help from a pastor, a doctor, a book? "I went to the Christian bookstore trying to find a book to help me," he said in a slow southern-Indiana drawl. "There just wasn't anything. So I finally bought a book on cancer, but it didn't help much. Is there anything you can tell me that might help?"

I stopped for a moment and thought about the fact that I now had five years of chronic illness "under my belt." I had some very basic coping techniques down, having been through a very private, personal hell – having stared death down and won, for the time being. I had come to terms with my illness in context to my relationship with the Lord. Where should I begin?

My heart went out to him, and I spent the next hour and a half trying to reassure him, giving him practical suggestions, and telling him that I truly cared.

A few days after the phone call, I wrote Tim a letter because my heart was heavy for him and I had thought of other things that I wished I would have shared with him. I am sharing the letter here with you, because it best sums up what I would say to you if we could sit down and have a heart to heart chat. Please keep in mind that I was only able to write this letter after five years of the pain and struggle to come to terms with an incurable illness.

Dear Tim,

I have not been able to get you out of my mind ever since our phone conversation. My heart goes out to you, and I am lifting your needs on wings of prayer to our all-powerful Lord who loves you immensely. Be assured that he knows every sigh that escapes you, every question, every doubt, every pain. He is totally in control of your situation and is ready to bring victory to you through it. I'm not saying that it's going to be easy, and it most definitely will not be quick. This is going to be the hardest battle you will ever wage against Satan, as he is prowling outside your doorstep right now plotting your defeat.

The insidious thing about a chronic illness is that it diverts your entire attention to your body, and you don't realize that your spirit is being destroyed. Your faith, your friendships, your sanity – everything is on the line right now. Don't cave in! You will feel like God is a million miles away. You will feel betrayed by your body. Hopelessness will begin to creep in and will take up permanent residency if you let it. Being told you have an incurable illness is a cold, hard slap in the face. Your inner man will want to fight, retaliate and get the upper hand. But fighting *always* makes us weaker. And in this case, you're fighting yourself. It won't work. I tried for a very long time.

Picture for a moment that you came down with a disease that paralyzed you from the waist down. That would be fact. You could point to it, see it, show it to your friends and relatives. Would you go out and sign up to run the Boston marathon? No. You'd get yourself a super-duper wheelchair and have a ramp built to your front door. The problem with most chronic illnesses is that there's nothing to point at and nothing for people to see. It's a silent, infuriating, invisible thing that nobody understands, least of all the patient. Give it time. Try to stop kicking and screaming inside at the rotten deal that it is. We are not the first people to come down with a life-changing disease – we just always thought it would happen to "somebody else." Not us! And especially not in the prime of our lives.

It might help to realize that most chronically ill people say that

19

the first year is the worst. Your body is reeling form the shock of the disease and it needs time to regroup its defenses. Try to be patient and hold on to the belief that it *will* get better. But very, very slowly.

It may be a long time before you can accept the reality of disease in your life. That's normal. But fighting it won't change anything, at least not physically. What you *can* fight are Satan, and feelings of helplessness, overwhelming despair, hopelessness, anxiety, anger, and fear for the future.

Remember, God is still in control. And yes, He does allow putrid, disgusting events to shape our lives and mold us into the faithful servants He wants us to be. That doesn't mean He loves us any less. A pastor once told me that God only gives assignments like this to the ones He is sure can handle it. Sometimes that doesn't feel like much of an honor, though. But He's watching and waiting to see if we're made of the stuff He hoped we were.

It took a long, long time, but I found out that I am, through His grace. It has been the most difficult experience I could have ever imagined, but I have come out on the other side with a totally new faith and a new understanding of what Jesus did for me on the cross. Jesus Himself felt all of our feelings of anger, betrayal, loneliness, fear and confusion. He really does understand. And in time, it is my prayer that you will find other Christians who can help you bear your burden. . . .

It was this phone call and others like it that prompted me to write this book. I am not a doctor or a psychologist, but I am somebody who has lived with a chronic, incurable illness for five and a half years now. There were days when I just plain wanted to die and get it over with.

I didn't know anyone else who had ever been told that they weren't going to die – but never get well. I didn't know where to turn for help, who to talk to. My pastor had never before counselled someone in my position, and he seemed uncomfortable and embarrassed. In short he said, "I don't know what to say to you. But if you ever get to the place where you're ready to turn your back on Jesus, let me know."

I searched Christian bookstores for a book to help me, as my friend Tim had. I found books on death and dying, and terminal illness, but nothing for me, personally, written by someone who had "been there."

THE SEARCH FOR A DIAGNOSIS

If you have been diagnosed with a chronic illness or disability, the word "incurable" is probably the scariest thing you have ever heard uttered in your life. It feels like someone has thrown a bowling ball at the pit of your stomach. Your thoughts and feelings are reeling, tumbling out of control with questions like, "Why me?" "How am I ever going to learn to live with this?" and, "How will my family deal with this?"

You are probably feeling angry, depressed and relieved all at the same time, because most chronically ill people struggle to obtain a diagnosis for a long time before one finally comes through. Once it does, we're not sure if we're glad or not.

Or maybe they haven't been able to pin a "label" on you yet. Realize that doctors are not God and just because they can't substantiate what you're feeling doesn't mean it's not really there, or that you're crazy. Believe in yourself, and be gentle with yourself. A diagnosis will come in time.

Kathleen Lewis, a registered nurse, says in her book, *Successful Living with Chronic Illness*: "Until you are diagnosed, you may have had serious doubts about your sanity. Doubts of this nature may have been voiced by a physician or two along the way, as well as by family and friends.

"Up to this point, your experiences of your internal reality, *being sick*, may not have been verified or validated in your *external reality*. When the experiences of the outside world and the inside world don't correlate, you have a unique type of insanity, all by itself. Diagnosis may bring a meshing of the two. Then again, your worst fears may be realized, putting your sanity to yet another test.[2]

One C.E.B.V. patient said, "As much as I hated hearing the doctor say, 'You have an incurable illness,' it was a turning point for me. I could no longer deny there was something wrong with me, and neither could my family. We had to face it, and once we did that, we were able to get on with our lives."

I, myself, struggled for two long years to obtain a diagnosis, in the midst of everyone thinking I was crazy. I could read it on their faces. I even began to wonder myself. I went to doctors from one end of the country to the other, spending thousands of dollars, waiting, waiting. Come on, Lord, I thought. If I had to get sick, couldn't it at least be something normal?

I have since found out, in talking with other chronically ill people, that all of my reactions were common. Many people who become chronically ill have never heard of their illness before, or if they have, they know little or nothing about it. Incurable illnesses and debilitating disabilities are something that happen to "other people." We rarely take the time to find out about something until it affects our personal lives very deeply. Five years ago I did not know a single chronically ill or disabled person. Now my life is filled with them. Funny how life has a way of involving us with people most like ourselves.

Before a diagnosis, our anxieties and fears about the unknown "it" are multiplied one-hundred fold. A diagnosis lets us get a handle on where we're at and where we're going. Instead of mumbling unintelligibly when someone asks what's wrong with us, we can speak up and say plainly, "I have. . . ."

I felt so free and relieved when the diagnosis finally came through, knowing that I didn't have to hide anymore. It also gave me the freedom to look at myself in a new light, one in which I didn't have to "pretend" to be well anymore, because the medical community had finally acknowledged that I *wasn't*.

THE MEANING OF CHRONIC ILLNESS

Most people are familiar with *acute* illnesses – the patient either eventually gets well, or he dies. The very word "chronic" in "chronic illness" connotes negative things in people's minds, as in "chronic complainer" or, "chronically late." So someone chronically ill would seem to already have a strike or two against himself. A term I prefer which is offered by the medical community is *phasic illness*, and it applies to illnesses such as Systemic Lupus Erythematosus (SLE), Rheumatoid Arthritis (RA), Multiple Sclerosis (MS) and Chronic Epstein-Barr Virus (C.E.B.V.), which is what I have. The patient has a waxing and waning of symptoms, daily ups and downs, or "phases" that he finds himself in.

Phasic illnesses are the least understood by society because there is nothing for people to *see* – the illness is painfully invisible, and we as patients have to fight every step of the way for credibility.

500,000 Americans are believed to have Multiple Sclerosis, 1 million, Lupus; 4 million, C.E.B.V; 36 million, arthritis; 12 million, severe asthma. And then there are those with debilitating heart disease, migraine and "cluster" headaches, and the millions from 18-40 who suffer from T.M.J. (temporomandibular jaw stress dysfunction) – all very real and debilitating, but which healthy people never stop to think about.[3]

The disabled of society, victims of car accidents, skiing accidents, and work-related accidents; polio patients, Vietnam Vets, and those born with genetic disorders, are more visible, but equally misunderstood. Here, also, there is no comfort in numbers. Over 1,000 Americans are severely hurt in accidents every hour, with a yearly toll of about 350,000 victims with one out of six adults between the ages of 18-64 are disabled due to accident or chronic illness.[4]

A person who awakens one day to find himself chronically ill or disabled goes into shock, retreats; then emerges slowly back into the "real world." His entire world has collapsed: financially, emotionally, physically, mentally and socially. Re-entry must be handled with the utmost care. Chronic illness and disability also reach out and grab the lives of loved ones and friends, leaving them frustrated and angry at their inability to help or truly understand.

The patient finds himself in the midst of several battles. Spiritually, he battles feelings of betrayal, hopelessness; feelings that God doesn't love him anymore or has forgotten about him. Emotionally, he battles losses of independence, financial freedom, spontaneity and childlike responses and pleasures. Physical losses include mobility, recreation and exercise, and freedom from pain and discomfort. And then there is the loss of role identity: usually a major vocational change takes place as the patient comes to grips with the inability to function in his old job and readjusts to a new set of circumstances, or perhaps finds himself discharged from the work force permanently.

One Lupus patient, a legal aide, said, "I was just sure that once I gave up working, I would go into remission. After all, I wouldn't have the stress of my job anymore, I could rest when I needed to – I was bound to get better, right?" When that didn't happen, the patient felt cheated and let down.

Kathleen Lewis, the registered nurse, says in *Successful Living with Chronic Illness* that adjustment to a chronic illness is 10 percent physical and 90 percent mental.[5] From a medical standpoint, perhaps, this is true. But for a Christian, I believe that the figures must be reevaluated to circumscribe just how much of the battle is spiritual.

And so, we will view chronic illness and disability in three ways throughout this book: first of all, our human reaction to it. Secondly, what the psychological and medical fields have to say on the subject, and lastly, what God's Word says to us to strengthen and encourage us.

OUR HUMAN REACTION: "WHY ME, LORD?"

My husband and I had gone back to our home town to attend a wedding, and there we ran into an old friend. She was the person who had introduced us to each other, and she had stood up for *our* wedding, but we hadn't been in touch for a long time now. I had heard that she had been having a lot of health problems, and during the reception, she told me about it. There were lots of female problems – endometrioses, an ovary removed, and finally, a complete hysterectomy in a young woman who was only 33 years old and still single. The worst part, she said, was that none of this had solved her problems, as her doctors assured her it would. She still had too many "vague" health problems – she was "chronically ill," but as yet, had no diagnosis.

After returning home, I received this letter:

Dear Cyndi,
There have been so many times in the past month that I've thought of you and your struggle with your health. I've been in

and out of the hospital and more doctor's offices than I care to think about since I saw you. There have been mysterious infections and lots of allergy problems, and lots of doctors who don't seem to quite know what to do. Tomorrow I go to an allergist/immunologist. Say a prayer for me, okay? I haven't been able to work or do much else, my finances are a disaster – but I am determined to deal with all of this. People have a hard time understanding my single-mindness in trying to find answers, but I can't stop trying until I get well. I'm trying to be able to take care of myself and find my purpose here in this world. There are certainly days when it seems that it would just be easier to give up . . . but I have to believe that I won't be given anything that I can't handle. I have always believed that everything happens for a reason. I didn't mean to go on like this, but I know that you truly understand. . . .

In essence, the cry of her heart is, "Why me?" What is the purpose, what is the *reason*, why am I feeling no peace inside? And then there are her words, "There certainly are days when it seems that it would just be easier to give up. . . . "

> I'm scared.
> So scared I can't think.
> I can't breathe.
> I can't move.
> If the doctors don't know what's wrong with me
>   then who does?
> If they told me I was going to die
>   I could face that.
> If they told me they had to operate
>   I could face that.
> But, they "*don't know*"?
>   Life is too short
> To be lived as one huge question mark.
>
>   C.M.

During the two years that I struggled along without a diagnosis – just day after day filled with unrelenting pain and hundreds of questions, I told the Lord that I would prefer to die, rather than deal with this daily and put my husband through it as well.

Death would have been the easy way out, from my seat on the boat. I could have gone straight to heaven, requested a conference with the Lord, and had all of my "Whys" neatly answered in a matter of minutes. I *wanted* to die, because I didn't know how I was going to face the future as a person who was constantly ill and in pain. And I certainly didn't want to inflict a future like that on my poor husband. Does it help you that I've shared that with you? I wish that someone would have shared it with me at the beginning of my illness, because I was ashamed of feeling that way. It seemed so weak and faithless.

Death is something that a non-Christian often doesn't want to discuss or even think about. But we as Christians usually have an exceedingly easier time with death, knowing that it's really a beginning rather than an end . . . a necessary plan carefully and lovingly constructed by the Father to bring His children to be with Him. It means an end to all suffering, pain and separation.

But chronic illness or disability is not the end to all suffering, it is only the beginning. And it does not put our hearts and minds to rest as death does, but instead stirs up heartfelt turmoil and hundreds of questions: "If the Lord really loves me, he wouldn't allow me to be incurably ill," we say. Or, "I've been a kind person and a good Christian. How can this be happening to me?" . . . "But the Bible says, 'Ask and you shall receive' and I've asked a hundred (or a thousand) times to be healed. Surely He will act soon."

Since the Lord had allowed a chronic illness into my life and not a terminal illness, I had to conclude that He had a reason for leaving me here, and I had to be content to wait until that reason was revealed. Job said, "If I die, I go out into the darkness, and call the grave my father and the worm my mother and my sister. Where then is my hope?" (Job 17:13-16 LB).

I was shocked at how quickly I would question God and ask "Why?" My immediate reaction was a feeling of betrayal – by my body, by my God. I was bitter and unyielding. I sulked and pouted and lashed out. I was near losing my mind.

What I was dealing with most of all was a collapse of my naive, childlike, complete and utter trust in the Lord . . . the belief that He would always take care of me. My faith was bruised. I felt helpless, hopeless and alone, and like God was on vacation. In Tahiti. And He wasn't taking any calls!

> Don't let your suffering embitter you at the one who can deliver you. Do you really think that if you shout loudly enough against God, he will be ashamed and repent? (Job 36:18,19 LB).

If you are reading this at a point where you are still asking "Why?" I'd like to remind you to be very patient and kind and gentle with yourself. Asking why is not a sign of weakness or a lack of faith – it's a sign that you're human. God made us "wonderfully and fearfully" (Psa. 139:14) and we are capable of great depth and understanding of the finer, more intricate points of God's Spirit when we commune with Him. But because of this, we sometimes forget that we really are weak, helpless creatures who are above all *human*.

We don't like "Whys" in life – or unanswered questions, or doubt, or fear. Unfortunately, chronic illness and disability encompass all of these and more: loss, grief and mourning, guilt, stress, intolerance, and credibility problems. And they're mentally, emotionally and spiritually draining. That's quite a lot to be dumped in our laps all at once.

In the midst of asking why and feeling betrayed and like the Lord just didn't love me anymore, one of the hardest things for me to face was that maybe the Lord had not in fact forgotten about me, but was behind my illness, having turned Satan lose in my life as He had Job's. How could this be? I had plans, big plans for my life. The Lord knew all about them, didn't He? Surely He wanted these enriching, wonderful things for my life. He couldn't possibly be allowing me to get sick and stay sick.

THE SOVEREIGNTY OF GOD

And then I came to the first and most critical step on the road to learning to live with an incurable illness. This was the concept of the *sovereignty of God.* He is God. The Great I AM. The Alpha and the Omega, the Beginning and End. And whether I like it or not, He *was* in control. I knew that in my head. I just didn't tend to like it much that He was actually going to step in and take control of my life.

Elizabeth Elliot, whose missionary husband was killed by savages said:

God is God. If it weren't for the sovereignty of God, I wouldn't be here. I wouldn't have anything to say, because the things that have happened to me have been shattering to any notion of what God is supposed to do. Again and again God has had to shake up my categories and strip away the veneers. He has had to remind me that my faith has to rest in who God *is*, not merely in what He does. *He is sovereign.* He says, 'I AM LORD.' That's a crucial question that has to be settled in the life of every individual at some time. When you study the biographies in the Bible, you see the endless suffering that God has had to put people through, and the lengths to which God would go to isolate a man and say to him in that silence, "I am the Lord." God has had to say that to me in each crisis.

Everything in our lives comes through the sovereign permission of a sovereign God, and this is never so clearly illustrated as it is in the book of Job. It was always easy for me, before I became ill, to look a this lesson as a "nice story," and to say, "Three cheers for Job. The Lord allowed Him to be tested and he passed, and in the end God made it up to him by giving him back twice what he'd had in the beginning" (Job 42:10).

But that was before suffering had entered my life that no amount of prayer was taking away. That was before, I too, was ready to "curse God and die" (Job 2:9).

Job was stricken with sore boils from the "sole of his foot unto his crown" (Job 2:7 KJ). But this came only after he had lost all of his sheep and herdsmen and cattle and servants *and* all of his children. Suddenly it was no longer just a story to me. I put myself in Job's position and pictured myself with my illness – then pictured everything I owned and loved and cared about destroyed around me.

The Bible was my instruction manual for life – and there it was in black and white: If the Lord had *allowed* this in Job's life, then He certainly could *allow* something like my illness in my life.

GOD'S PURPOSE AND PLAN

God had a purpose and plan in Job's life and this was accomplished through pain and destruction. God had a purpose and plan in Joseph's life when He allowed Joseph to be sold into slavery by his brothers. Later on Joseph said to them, "As far as I am concerned, God turned into good what you meant for evil, for He brought me to this high position I have today so that I could save the lives of many" (Gen. 50:20, LB).

Life is not fair, nor is it just, but God is. Perhaps if you are fifty-years wise, you already knew that, and are handling your illness or disability fairly well. My problem was that I was 26 years old and no horrifically bad thing had ever happened to me before. I was pretty much unscathed by the fiery darts of soul-wrenching pain, and so when the illness struck, I cried "Foul!" and waited impatiently for the referee to charge out and penalize the other team.

We have that choice in the game of life – when things don't go our way, we can storm off the court, we can pout, we can shout at the referee. . . .

I waited for nothing, of course, and have since come to realize that loss, pain, sacrifice, and the forfeit of one's rights are really what life on earth is all about, just as sacrifice was the purpose of Jesus' life here on earth. It is beauty and hope and joy that are the rare, fleeting gifts, the jewels that we must treasure in our hearts while we have them.

The fact that the Lord has a purpose and a plan is a truth that we may not be able to easily accept, but it is truth.

> For my thoughts are not your thoughts, neither are my ways your ways, saith the Lord. For as the heavens are higher than the earth, so are my ways higher than your ways, and my thoughts than your thoughts (Isa. 55:8 KJ).

Nothing could have looked bleaker to the Christians of the time than the Son of God hanging on a cross. John W. Stott shares in his book, *The Cross of Christ*:

> The cross of Christ is the proof of God's solidary love, that of his personal, loving solidarity with us in our pain. For the real sting of suffering is not the misfortune itself, or even the pain or the injustice of it, but the apparent God-forsakenness of it. Pain is endurable, but the seeming indifference of God is not. Sometimes we picture him lounging, perhaps dozing, in some

celestial deck chair, while the hungry millions starve to death. We think of Him as an armchair spectator, almost gloating over the world's suffering, and enjoying His own insulation from it.

It is this terrible caricature of God which the cross smashes smithereens. We are not to envisage Him on a deck chair, but on a cross. The God who allows us to suffer, once suffered Himself in Christ, and continues to suffer with us and for us today.

Since the cross was a once-for-all historical event, in which God in Christ bore our sins and died our death because of His love and justice, we must not think of it as expressing an eternal sinbearing in the heart of God. What Scripture does give us warrant to say, however, is that God's eternal, holy love, which was uniquely exhibited in the sacrifice of the cross, continues to suffer with us in every situation in which it is called forth.[6]

FACT, NOT FEELINGS

We have to make the choice, in our pain, to go with what we *know*, rather than what we feel. Scripture invites us to look at what we *know* in regard to our suffering:

We also rejoice in our sufferings, because we *know* that suffering produces perseverance; perseverance, character; and character, hope (Rom. 5:3,4 NIV).

And also in James it tells us:

Consider it joy, my brothers, whenever you face trials of many kinds, because you *know* that the testing of your faith develops perseverance. Perseverance must finish its work so that you may be mature and complete, not lacking anything (James 1:2-4 NIV).

Truth is truth, and God's truth doesn't change. He is the same "yesterday, today, and tomorrow" (Hebrews 13:8). Satan wants to control our emotions, and so make us *think* God's truth changes acording to our circumstances.

God is, above everything else, *good*. We must cling to that truth. God cannot do anything contrary to the nature of His character, and all that He permits to come into our lives must be intrinsic with His nature.

> And we know that all things work together for good to them that love God and are called according to His purpose (Rom. 8:28 KJ).

> Taste and see that the Lord is good: blessed is the man that trusteth in Him (Psa. 34:8).

We *know* also that God is powerful, just, "Shall not the Judge of all the earth do right?" (Gen. 18:25 KJ); holy, and that He has total knowledge. "But the very hairs of your hair are numbered, fear ye not . . ." (Matt. 10:30,31 KJ).

Sometimes important spiritual truths are easier to accept as "head-knowledge" than they are as "heart-knowledge." Knowing something is true in our *hearts* takes time, but if we give it time and are patient and prayerful, God has a chance to work. If we shut God's truth out, we shut God out.

There is great freedom in acknowledging God's sovereignty and accepting a divine plan for illness in our lives. It allows us to move beyond the question of "Why me?" and onto the business of learning to live with an incurable illness or disability.

We will continue to look at God's plan for our illness, His purpose in trials, and the spiritual battle that Satan tries to wage against us in our illness in the following chapters.

Endnotes

1. Franklin Shontz, *The Psychological Aspects of Physical Illness and Disability,* (Macmillan, 1975), pp. 112-113.

2. Lewis, Kathleen, *Successful Living with Chronic Illness,* (Wayne, N.J.: Avery Publishing Group, 1985), p. 73.

3. Figures from: The National Multiple Sclerosis Society, The Lupus Foundation of America, The National C.E.B.V. Syndrome Association, Contra Costa (CA). *Times,* 6 Sept., 1989, The American Lung Association, The TMJ Foundation.

4. National Safety Council, Accident Facts, (Washington, D.C.: NSC, 1978). U.S. Bureau of the Census, Statistical Abstract of the U.S.: 1982-83, (Washington, D.C.: Gov't. Printing Office, 1982).

5. Lewis, p. 135

6. Stott, John, *The Cross of Christ,* (Intervarsity Press, 1986).

2

THE MENTAL AND EMOTIONAL BATTLE

History books tell us that battles have rarely been won overnight. They require great mental, emotional and physical preparation, and many times months or even years before victory is achieved.

So why is it when we go into battle in the early stages of our illness or disability, we expect to walk away victorious with little or no effort? Is it because we have always felt in control of our bodies up until this point, and we're just sure that if we grit our teeth long enough, "This too, shall pass" and life will get back to normal?

For all of the people I interviewed for this book, the first stages of their illness or disability were the roughest. Judith O'Brien, a 50 year old Lupus patient, says she gave herself two months to "get over" Lupus, "or else." "Or else what?" I asked.

"I didn't know! I had just made up my mind that was all the time I was going to give it. Some days I would think, 'It's okay. I'm a strong person, I can handle anything.' The next day I would be back to 'Why me?' again. Two years later I was *still* thinking 'This IS going to go away!' "

We battle our minds and wills, which will not accept the reality of a permanent illness or disability. We battle feelings of helplessness and hopelessness that we see reflected in the eyes of loved ones and strangers alike. We are often battling the system for our rightful worker's compensation benefits, yet at the same time hating the thought of taking "welfare."

Life comes to screeching halt at the onset of a permanent illness or disability. As one sufferer says, "Chronic illness takes your life and smashes it against the wall." We are at first in shock that this is even happening to us. Then we begin to grope wildly for solutions and answers. When we reach the stone-cold truth that this is real and it is permanent, we may feel like crawling into bed and pulling the covers up over our heads and telling the world to go away. That's what Kathy Perdue, a 38-year old C.E.B.V. patient says she wanted to do:

But lying in bed is no fun, and I realized if I stayed there long enough, it could kill me. So I began fighting back.

When fighting back did no good, anger and resentment began welling inside me, as I realized that *I was expected to change.* Change is a part of life, but it took me over a year to realize that I had to admit I had something that was going to alter my lifestyle.

She went on to tell me,

I play a mental game with myself, which is self-defeating, saying to myself, "Maybe today it (her illness) will be gone." The problem is that normal illnesses have a definite progression, but this doesn't. I never know what kind of day it's going to be. I have "okay" days. I have what I call "pusher" days, when I have to push myself along all day to get anything accomplished. And then I have days when I simply cannot function.

I am constantly prioritizing. I pray and ask God, "Okay, so it's not going to be a good day. What should I do first?" And then about the time I feel I have that down pat, I start saying, "Okay, God, I've learned to prioritize and I've learned what's important. Can't you please take this illness from me now?"

These mental games that we play with ourselves are normal. Psychologists tell us that there are five stages or phases that a person goes through when he suffers a huge personal loss, whether it be personal, professional, physical, etc. They are called the five stages of grief, and they are classified as Denial, Anger, Bargaining, Depression, and Acceptance.[1] Perhaps you are already familiar with them, but I want to cover them in the aspects that they relate to chronic illness and disability. I was already familiar with these stages when I became ill, but I associated them only with grief from *death*. I was almost to the acceptance stage before I realized what I had been going through. These stages have also been expressed as Who, me? Not me! Why me? and Yes, me.

DENIAL

Everyone goes through these stages at a time of loss, though some people pass through them more quickly than others, and some might hit a stage such as denial or depression and be stuck there. My grandfather was operated on for prostate cancer five years ago. Even though he went through radiation treatments until he was considered permanently in remission, he still to this day vehemently denies that he ever had cancer. "Just an idea those stupid doctors got into their heads," he'll say, or, "Just another way for them to get into my wallet." He will probably deny it until the day he meets his Maker.

For those who have just been told they are incurably ill, *owning up to the truth* of it is the first step of many to getting on with life and restructuring it in a way in which we can learn to cope, some of us better than others.

Psychologist Franklin Shontz tells us about three types of denial in his book, *The Psychological Aspects of Physical Illness and Disability:*

> Purely *defensive* denial tends to expand progressively, so that more and more of the personality becomes dependent upon its maintenance. The longer one waits to break through such denial, the more difficult is the process and the more devastating are its effects. A person who puts up a bold, aggressive facade of unrealistic denial may be covertly developing resources for testing reality. He will not abandon his defense until he is sure that a positive approach stands a good chance of succeeding.

He goes on to discuss a second type, which he terms *marginality,* occurs when a person is caught between two identities; one he desires, but cannot possess (a healthy body), and one that is available but unacceptable (an unhealthy one). In illness and disability, marginality occurs because identity as a 'normal person' is positively valued, whereas identity as a 'helpless invalid' or cripple is repulsive."

And then there is a third type of behavior, similar yet different from denial. It is known as "as if" behavior. "A person who is desperately frightened of being recognized as ill or disabled may do all within his power to conceal it. This is based on the false premise that threat can be successfully avoided by acting as if it did not exist."[2] In other words, if we deny our illness and act as though it doesn't exist, maybe it will go away. This is the psychological equivalent of sweeping dirt under the carpet and saying the house is clean.

> Denial isn't all bad. I'm sick, but I keep going. I push away all the implications of my illness so I can function today. That's useful denial.[3]

During my phase of denial, my spiritual reaction was to delve into the Word, and I literally spent weeks, all day long, just reading what it had to say about healing. I read and read and I prayed and waited. And waited. And waited. I was just sure that God was going to heal me, because there are dozens of scriptures about healing, and I was "claiming" all of them, over and over, day after day.

During this time I learned a very important lesson: YOU CAN'T BEAT GOD OVER THE HEAD WITH HIS OWN WORD. Because for every scripture that we pull out and believe on and pray over, there is another scripture two books over that deals with the same issue from an entirely different perspective.

Does God's Word lie? Of course not. It's just that God has reserved the right of carrying out His perfect will in all believers' lives, and when we became believers, *we gave Him that right.* Now that we're sick, are we going to renege? Paul may have wanted to scream, "Lord, this isn't fair!" when he received the "thorn" in his side. He knew that Jesus had brought Lazarus back to life, he knew about all the healings that Jesus had performed. He could have easily jutted out his bottom lip, pointed to these things and cried, "But, Lord!"

And yet, what did Jesus say of Paul in Acts 9:15, right after Paul had been struck blind and been without food and water for three days? "Paul is my chosen instrument, to take my message to the nations and before kings, as well as to the people of Israel. *And I will show him how much he must suffer for me.*" It was Jesus' plan, carefully mapped out, that Paul suffer! And shortly after, the Word tells us, "Paul became more and more fervent in his preaching." His suffering only fueled his faith.

> And since we are his children, we will share his treasures – for all God gives to his Son Jesus is now ours, too. But if we are to share his glory, we must also share his suffering. Yet what we suffer now is nothing compared to the glory he will give us later. For all creation is waiting patiently and hopefully for that future day when God will resurrect his children. For on that day, thorns and thistles, sin, death and decay – the things that overcame the world against its will at God's command – will all disappear, and the world around us will share in the glorious freedom from sin which God's children enjoy. For we know that even the things of nature, like animals and plants, suffer in sickness and death as they await this great event. And even we Christians, although we have the Holy Spirit within us as a foretaste of future glory, also groan to be released from pain and suffering. We, too, wait anxiously for that day when God will give us our full rights as his children, including the new bodies that He had promised us, *bodies that will never be sick again* and will never die (Rom. 8:17-23 LB).

And so, I had to ask myself, was I willing to suffer for Jesus, even just a little bit? Denying my illness wasn't going to make it go away. Refusing to accept it just because the scriptures tell of specific incidents when it was God's perfect will to heal someone did not mean that it was His perfect will in my life. Paul said, "Three different times I begged him to make me well again. Each time He said, 'No, I am with you. That is all you need. My power shows up best in weak people' " (I Cor. 12:8,9 LB).

After a period of denial because I "knew" that God was

going to heal me, and He didn't, I was still wanting to regress to childhood, that magical time of life when my parents could make everything all better by a simple kiss and a pat. And after awhile when I got good and tired of waiting and waiting and waiting for the Lord to act, I got angry.

ANGER

And maybe that is where you are right now – hurt and resentment and bewilderment and anxiety have escalated themselves into a full head of angry steam, so much of it that you don't know what you're going to do with it all and you feel you're going to explode.

You're angry for having an illness – but whom should you be angry at – God, fate, the whole world? You're angry at doctors because they have no cure for your disease. You thought doctors knew so much, but now you realize they don't. You're angry at family members and friends who are at times unavailable when you need them, and expect more of you than you can do. You wish they could live in your body for a day or even an hour so they could understand what life is like for you. Then maybe they wouldn't say or do things that hurt your feelings. You're also upset by the thought that they might resent all they have to do for you – and you feel hurt and resentful in return.

If you have a disability that requires you to rely on others for your daily needs, you're constantly frustrated. You're frustrated because you can't do these things for yourself, and you're frustrated because others don't do them promptly enough or exactly as you would like. It also frustrates and angers you to be unable to engage in activities in which you once took pride.[4]

Anger may be evoked by healthy people, since they are a reminder of what has been lost. Healthy people handling minor health problems in an irresponsible manner may cause you to steam. The chronically ill may have to suffer silently, sharing their trials with only a "special few."

The inability of the "crowd" to "listen" may provoke anger. Fear of losing the support of significant others and your inability to function may generate anger. The need for others to deny your illness can be maddening – "You *look* so good!"

There may be anger and resentment on the part of the person who has your dependency needs thrust on him. You may experience more anger and frustration when only marginally ill than when severely ill, since you may have one foot in the world of the healthy and one foot in the world of the sick. You can't be totally in either world.[5]

Dr. Franklin Shontz goes on to say:

> In human beings, emotions are subtle and not directly tied to action. This is especially the case in physical illness: it cannot be attacked because it is intangible. The sick person may be intensely angry at the virus that "laid him low," but there is little he can do about it directly. For him, the equivalent of direct action is a kind of impotent rage, which he may vent on himself or on the nearest bystander (perhaps a nurse) for lack of a more suitable target. The person with a permanent disability may turn his anger toward his own helplessness into aggressive determination to overcome his limitations by hard work in rehabilitation. Some sick people turn anger outward, blaming others for their illness or their failure to improve. Others turn anger inward, blaming themselves for their condition and feeling guilty because they cause themselves and others so much trouble and expense.[6]

What should you do with all of this frustration and anger? Consider and understand, as best you can, the feelings and circumstances of the other person before expressing your anger. Knowing when and how to express anger is the key. Just because it is sometimes correct to let it out doesn't mean that it is always correct.[7] It might help immensely just to get alone by yourself and just go ahead and explode! Take your bed pillow and beat it viciously against the bed until you feel a release. Or as soon as everyone is out of the house, yell your head off. Shout to the heavens and tell the Lord how you feel: hurt, put-upon, betrayed, seething, fearful, hopeless, lost, abused, and forgotten.

But hold it right there. Has the guilt set in yet? Aren't Christians supposed to be "first of all pure and full of quiet gentleness" (James 3:17)? Aren't the fruits of the Spirit ripe with peace, patience, and self-control (Gal. 5:22)?

Yes. But now we are back to the issue of our humanness. And humans, like animals, respond to pain in a very basic, unlovely, often unholy manner. We have the flesh waging its particular type of war while the spirit cries out in the midst of its war. Our two main goals should be:

IGNORE THE RAGING FLESH
and
CONTROL THE RAGING SPIRIT.

One of the most basic reasons that a life-changing illness or disability is so hard to bear is because we have always felt in control of our bodies and our lives. We have suffered from "ownership of self"[8] and we get angry when we realize that we do *not* in fact own ourselves, and are not in control of the situation. We do not own ourselves because we have been bought with a price by the Lord Himself with the blood of our precious Savior.

When we take on ownership of self, we become responsible for how life should come out. But we are a finite in a bewildering and infinite creation, and so we are lost.

It's a fact that we become emotionally possessive of the things we own. We are emotionally bothered when our property is lost, damaged or stolen. I had two suitcases stolen in New York City, and it took a year to find the perfect shade of peach blouse to go with the skirt I'd left at home . . . the jewelry was of sentimental value only and could never be replaced – and then there was the Bible I'd had since the day I'd gotten saved. It was dog-eared and falling apart, but it meant everything to me. These losses bothered me *a lot.*

The point is how much more possessive we feel over our own bodies, which we consider "ours" and have had since birth. We have no control over them now that they are sick and weak and unyielding. How dare they!

I have to admit that losing control over my body made me angrier than anything else when I realized I was incurably ill. I was always strong-willed and determined, and anything I set my mind to, I achieved. For someone who measured her self-worth by how much I physically accomplished in a day, I was in BIG trouble, because I could no longer control it. I couldn't even get out of bed, let alone accomplish everything on my ever-present "list." And realizing that I was no longer in control meant the reality of having to accept help.

Wait a minute! I was the one with the shoulder people cried on, always ready to sit and listen, hold a hand, wipe a tear. I was the one who made meals and baked cookies for people. I was the helper, not The Helpless One. And suddenly I hated myself and the role I was being forced to play. Self-esteem went out the window and guilt flew in.

Loss of control, loss of self-respect, loss of privacy – the theme of loss and betrayal became my focus. I became touchy, irritable, resentful. I cried until I felt I had used up every teardrop allotted in the universe, and then I cried some more.

It is possible that instead of venting our anger and letting it out of our systems, we let it fester and begin to close God out. We need to tell Him that we're angry, but then we need to ask Him to take that anger away. We have to reach a certain maturity in our walk with the Lord as we do in everyday life – eventually there comes a time when we stop throwing temper tantrums (at least for most of us!) and we come to see that talking quietly and honestly to our parents gets us much further than ranting and raving. It's amazing to see the difference in their response to us. And I believe that God breathes a sigh of relief when we stop exhibiting such childlike behavior with him. Bring a cup of coffee to the table, sit down across from Him, and say, "Okay, I've been behaving like a spoiled brat. Can we discuss this like adults?" Eventually that still, small voice will speak.

What I finally came back to was the issue of the sovereignty of God. Who was I to be angry with God, or angry with the way my life was coming out?

> Yet, O Lord, you are our Father. We are the clay, you are the potter, we are all the work of your hand (Isa. 64:8 NIV).

> But who are you, O man, to talk back to God? Shall what is formed say to him who formed it, "Why did you make me like this?" (Rom. 9:20 NIV).

Lloyd H. Ahlem talks about the concept of "ownership of self" in his book, *How to Cope With Conflict, Crisis, and Change:*

> How different for the one who believes fully that he is not his own, but is possessed by another – the living God. He has willingly turned over the title of himself to God. Then there is no more to protect, so no loss need be suffered. One day we are

45

going to turn it all over to God anyway, so why not do it willing-
ly now? Someone has said that we are born without our
consent and we die against our will, but between these events
we act as if we are ours by our own choosing. I believe it was
Bishop James Pike who said that being a Christian means dying
once so we won't have to do it again.[9]

BARGAINING

Perhaps you'll have knowing, caring people come to you
and tell you that you're sick or you've had this accident because
of a sin problem in your life. Now, only you know if this is true,
and a time of self-examination is a good thing, in fact, a necessary thing. But don't self-examine yourself to death. If there's
sin, get rid of it. Search your heart for any deep, secret sins,
and confess any unconfessed sins. Then get on with the business of learning to cope. Don't get hung up on "If I give this
up, Lord, will you make me well?" Acknowledge that there's a
purpose for your illness or injury and don't drive yourself crazy
with the "what -abouts." And don't make any rash promises
you'll regret – "If you make me well, Lord, I'll go be a missionary to the cannibals." He might just take you up on it, and you
might decide you'd rather have stayed sick!

I think bargaining is lessened for the mature Christian. As a
result, he gets to the resolution more quickly. He realizes he
lives in an economy of grace, not of bargaining. He has what
he has by the grace of God. Therefore, if he loses something,
that is also within the providence of His grace. God owned it
anyway. But he also knows that he really is in no position to
bargain with God. Keeping a bargain made with God is only re-
peating an atonement already accomplished. It is trying to earn
what has already been freely given.[10]

Once again, God is God. He has a perfect will for us and there is not one thing we can add to that, nor can we change God's view on the subject.

> Oh, what a wonderful God we have! How great are his wisdom and knowledge and riches! *How impossible it is for us to understand his decisions and methods.* For who among us can know the mind of the Lord? Who knows enough to be his counselor and guide? *And who could ever offer to the Lord enough to induce him to act?* For everything comes from God alone. Everything lives by his power, and *everything* is for his glory (Rom. 11:33-36, LB, emphasis mine).

Isn't that beautiful? God told us this to put our minds at ease. *Everything* is for His glory, even sickness and disability.

DEPRESSION

Once you're through with the senseless business of bargaining with God and you've worked through your anger and denial, you'll probably feel like you've been thrown into a pit of despair that you'll never be able to climb out of. Things may seem their bleakest now because you feel like you've run out of useful emotion and viable options. Depression sets in. Guilt and fear and mourning and stress make up your days. Your natural response may be to isolate yourself from the outside world, thinking they'll never understand. By avoiding people, you're also subconsciously insulating yourself from further hurt and pain. It's easy now to fall into the trap of fearing further disillusionment, thereby becoming cynical about life, or snide. You may become touchy, sharp, bitter – bewildering and hurting those around you who love you and are desperately trying to understand, although, "No one could possibly understand how I feel" is what you're probably telling yourself over and over.

The truth of the matter is that you're right. Someone who has never had the "sentence" of chronic illness pronounced over their head *can* never know exactly what you're going through – but they can try. And if they're truly a good friend, steadfast family member, or devoted spouse, they *will, if you let them.* And that means not pushing them away with one hand while trying to draw them near for comfort with the other.

I spent so much time ranting and raving, fluctuating between anger and depression for so long, that I thought for sure I was going to drive my husband of six years away for good. I would scream and cry until I was exhausted – trying to flush the demons of despair from my soul, perhaps secretly wishing that he *would* go away, and then I wouldn't have to feel guilty for "ruining his life" anymore. But once I would stop ranting and sink into a numbing, bone-chilling, steely-eyed depression, I would find he was still there, in love, taking me firmly by the shoulders and saying sternly, "You have got to get a grip on yourself. You have *got* to stop feeling sorry for yourself." Which would, of course, at times make me all the angrier or more depressed. He had a point, though. From a psychologist's standpoint, depression is often just glamorized self-pity. And why do we get depressed? Because *our* plans go awry, *our* health is suddenly taken from us, *our* bodies hurt and pain us, *our* freedom and independence are limited.

Rather narrow vision, all this focusing on Me and Myself, isn't it? And yet, when we turn our focus completely inward, depression is going to result.

A period of depression is completely normal, and in fact, necessary. The only healthy reaction to many life situations is depression, and it is a common psychological response to stress.[11] Depression at least means that we've moved on from the denial stage, although some people fluctuate between the two for a period of time. It is estimated that even healthy people are depressed 40 percent of the time, just from stress and trying to cope with day to day living.[12]

What is really happening at the first pangs of depression is the beginning of the grief process. Did you think, as I did, that grieving only took place when someone died? But you see, if you are chronically ill or disabled, someone *has* died – the *old you.* And you are going to grieve and mourn and be broken-hearted for the "you" that you used to be: alive, vibrant, independent, HEALTHY. One amputee who lost his leg said, "I used to practice at the hospital getting used to my new leg by going up and down steps. But there were no exercises to practice letting go of the person I used to be."

You are going to grieve for all the future hopes and plans you had saved up and stored in a corner of your heart. You're going to grieve for your family and friends and spouse because of what you feel you're "putting them through." You're going to grieve for your children and feel guilty because you can no longer hope of being a model parent who goes out roller skating, sledding, or playing baseball with them. You're going to grieve for your relationship with the Lord, because you will never again enjoy the childlike, innocent trust that you had "pre-illness."

Your spouse and family will be going through their own grief processes. People go through these stages at different paces, and if someone reaches a level before the other person achieves it, problems can rapidly arise. Says Kathy Perdue, the C.E.B.V. patient, who used to strive to be "super-Mom": "I have to fight to be the person my husband married, and that takes a lot of energy, which just weakens me. He grieves for the person I used to be."

From now on, your entire life will be, consciously, or unconsciously, divided into two categories: PRE-ILLNESS and POST-ILLNESS.

GRIEF AND MOURNING

In looking at grief and mourning, it helps to look at the "little deaths" that occur along the way in life. The process is slow and painful.

One can understand this notion by recalling the many dyings one experiences along the way to one's final death: the dying of one's youthful self as the natural aging process occurs; the loss of friends through death, moves, and changes in interests; the death of one's identity as another emerges (divorce and retirement are two prime examples.) Disappointment can be seen as a type of little death. "I was crushed," we say, or "It fell through,"or "It was a shattering blow." All these expressions use powerful death imagery. . . . How do we respond to these little deaths? What are the key factors in accepting their inevitability and their power to change our lives? How do we hope others will respond to them? . . . No more powerful example of a person's sudden confrontation with a little death exists than the experience of disabling illness or injury. Such a person abruptly, often unwillingly, but inevitably learns what it means to have "died." The little death might be as dramatic a dying in the eyes of the world as the young athlete who dies to hopes of Olympic stardom, or as unheralded as the young father who dies to the possibility of ever again taking his child for a walk in the woods.[13]

Psychologists tell us that mourning is a sudden destructuring of the life situation, loss of boundaries, and disintegration of organization. The more complete the destructuring, the more intense the mourning. As necessary as it is when loss occurs, mourning is not by itself productive. The positive functions mourning serves are to drain off undirected tension and to prepare for later reconstruction of psychological organization.[14]

Isolating ourselves during mourning is a natural defense mechanism against further pain and disillusionment. We feel that we're handling all we can right now, thank you, and we'd just rather be left alone.

SELF-PITY

But while we're off in a corner licking our wounds and trying to regroup, a dastardly little demon can sneak in the back door, and it's called self-pity. *It's the most destructive thing that can be allowed into our lives at this point,* a hundred times more destructive than our illness or disability itself. We have to be on the watch for it and instantly reevaluate ourselves and our position with it. Dr. Leslie Parrot, in his book, *The Habit of Happiness*, (Word Books, 1987), tells of Prof. Ernest O. Milby of Michigan State University, who used to tell his students that no one can be an effective marriage partner, parent, or employee if he has to take on the emotional overload of self-pity. (Let me add to that list "effective Christian"). Again and again, Prof. Milby warned his students, "Self-pity is the luxury that you cannot afford."

The probabilities are that most people will go through life with some key problem unresolved. Some will understand this and not permit the negative emotions to grow. Others will nourish their resentments with self-pity until they have distorted their personalities and become hating, hostile, difficult people.[15]

Imagine a couple whose little boy is run over by a car and killed. They stop communicating as each withdraws into his or her own grief, yet they refuse to seek counseling. They become mad at the world and mad at God, and the husband begins drinking. Twenty years later, their family is in shambles. This is self-pity in living color, and it's heart-wrenching.

During the time that you are caught up in the throes of depression and self-pity, you may slowly begin to lose your grip on reality altogether, and feel, either mildly or strongly, that you are losing your mind.

I first began to experience this during the time when I was still questioning and searching for the *reasons* for my illness. God seemed so very far away. I was convinced He was on vacation and told everyone so. And then some well-meaning but misguided people began pressuring me about divine healing. I had attended a "healing service," believing fully that God would work a miracle. Here is what I recorded in my journal the next day, my writing floating hazily over the pages, unlike my normal writing at all:

Never before have I been driven so dangerously near the edges of insanity. I never wondered much what it would be like but supposed it felt as though one were going over an edge. But it does not – sanity appears as a big beautiful ocean and you find yourself drifting farther and farther out in circles and toward the shore – and suddenly you feel as though you're the tide and you're rippling in, lapping against the bank once, twice. . . . If you never flow back out from the shore, you're there forever. Faded away. Gone. This was how I felt driving home from the healing service. Dead silence in the car . . . rippling farther and farther out. And no one knew. . . . All I have is the Word. I can hardly believe that God can take me any deeper or test my faith any more, but He must have the strength ready to give me also. He has to have, because the natural man in me is ready to give up. No more seeking, no more pressure, no more trying to go deeper . . . It's just too painful. I want to rest in the Word, but I feel such turmoil. All I want to do is just cry and cry and cry. . . .

Keeping a journal might prove very beneficial to you during the grief process. Writing out your feelings can help you rid yourself of them, and you emerge clear-headed and with a more positive attitude. Writing your feelings out in a letter and sending it to a close family member, friend, or even your spouse might help understanding for both parties tremendously. One psychologist, in speaking about how chronically ill people handle depression, said there are two paths a person might be tempted to take. The first is suicide. This is effective in the elimination of pain, and it's also very effective in striking out at any and everybody you ever blamed for your illness. The problem, he says, is that the person is no longer around to "enjoy" the effect. The second path is what he referred to as "the gutter." This can take many forms: self-mutilation, alcoholism or drug addiction, perhaps committing a crime and being sent to prison, perhaps having an affair . . . any destructive behavior with far-reaching affects. "A person can slide past the point where nobody's ever going to be able to catch him," he said. "Nobody can – if he doesn't *want* to be caught. He has to make up his mind."

If you feel that depression has moved in and taken up permanent residency, counseling might not only be beneficial, but imperative. I firmly believe that God has all the answers, but I also believe that he gives each of us different insights into these answers. "Two are better than one . . . if one falls down, his friend can help him up" (Eccl. 4:9, LB). A counselor might be just the right neutral "friend" to help in times of trouble.

53

WE HAVE TO LOVE JESUS
MORE THAN WE LOVED OUR
HEALTH.

Since depression and grieving have us focusing our attention inward, our eyes are no longer on Jesus. "Keep your eyes on Jesus, our leader and instructor . . ." (Heb. 12:2, LB). We run a great risk of letting our health become our whole focus, our first love.

> Yet I hold this against you: you have forsaken your first love (Rev. 2:4, LB).

> Friendship with God is reserved for those who reverence him. With them alone he shares the secrets of his promises (Psa. 25:14, LB).

What we must come to terms with in our depression is the reality of death and resurrection in our lives. We are depressed because our former selves are gone and a type of death has taken place. But like the seed that is dropped into the ground and must die before it bursts forth with new life, we must put our old selves into the ground and let them die before we can become the "new us" that God intends and our illness or disability demands. And here we have our hope, our resurrection.

Lloyd H. Ahlem says in *How to Cope With Conflict, Crisis and Change:*

> Hope is the antithesis of self-pity. The two are incompatible mental roommates. Both are implicit belief statements. The man who hopes believes something positive. The self-pitier is a doubter. While suffering he uses self-pity to gain attention, reinforcing the tendency to self-pity. People recover from emotional problems more quickly when they consciously decide to cut short their self-pity. The person who is healing well emotionally

sees that he must choose between hope and pity and that his choice is an expression of what he truly believes in his heart. So he participates actively in his own reconstruction, carrying the initiative for progress, brushing off those who would feel sorry for him.[15]

We can begin to search out new paths or directions the Lord might be leading us down. Even a Christian who is physically incapacitated need never feel useless or uninvolved in the Lord's work.

In his book, *Keep on Keeping On*, Harold I. Fickett Jr. told about his call on a woman who had suffered a severe heart attack. Confined to her home, she was very discouraged. She complained to Pastor Fickett about her uselessness. Oh, how she wanted to do some meaningful work for the Lord! Fickett told her kindly that in her new situation she could minister with power. "You have no place to go. You can use your time in praying for God's servants all over the world. Begin by remembering me as your pastor before the throne of God, and then pray for all the Christian workers that you know." The woman followed her pastor's advice, and she found joy and a new sense of purpose in life.

Prayer for others, especially God's servants, is a much-needed ministry, and it's something every Christian can do. There's no reason that a shut-in has to feel shut out from the Lord's work.[16]

Endnotes

1. Kubler-Ross, Elizabeth, *On Death and Dying,* (N.Y. Macmillian, 1969), pp. 34, 44, 72, 75, 99.

2. Shontz, p. 147, 169, and Shontz citing B.A. Wright, *Physical Disability – A Psychological Approach,* (N.Y.: Harper and Row, 1960).

3. Chyatte, Samuel, M.D., *On Borrowed Time: Living With Hemodialysis,* (Oradell, N.J., Medical Economics, 1979), p 10.

4. Flapan, Mark, PhD., "Living With a Rare Disorder – Feelings I Keep to Myself," *Nord,* Vol. 5, No.3.

5. Lewis, p. 53.

6. Shontz, p. 146

7. Lewis, p. 58, and Lewis citing Carter, L., *Good 'n' Angry,* (Grand Rapids, Michigan: Baker Book House, 1983), p.98.

8. Term coinage, Ahlem, Lloyd H., *How to Cope With Conflict, Crisis, and Change,* (Regal Books, G/L Publishing, 1978), p. 140.

9. Ibid. p 141

10. Ahlem, p. 50.

11. Flach, Fredric F., M.D., *The Secret Strength of Depression,* (Philadelphia: Lippincott, 1974), p, 16.

12. Lanier, B.G., "The Emotional and Psychological Aspects of Dealing With Systemic Lupus Erythematosus," speech given to the Greater Atlanta Chapter, Lupus Foundation of America, Inc., April 1981.

13. Purtillo, Ruth B., p. 280

14. Shontz, p. 170.

15. Ahlem, p. 86

16. R.W. DeHaan, "Shut in But Not Shut Out," *Our Daily Bread,* Vol. 34, Nos. 3, 4, 5, June, 1989.

3

AND FINALLY, ACCEPTANCE

A person can react in three different ways to a chronic illness: The first is to give up. The second is to fight it continually, which leads to despair. The third road is to get active on your own behalf and take responsibility for your well-being and your goals for the future.[1]

For the first year, *"I know I'm going to get well,"* played in my head like a warped record, occupying close to every second of my day.

By the second year, I had slumped dejectedly into knowing this was real – this was it. Now, just every once in a while, I get a flicker of hope . . . "Maybe." Maybe someday I'll have the energy to go back to school, start another business, hike, sing, run again! But that time is not now.

To everything there is a season, and a time for every purpose
under the heaven:
A time to be born, and a time to die; a time to plant and a time
to pluck up that which is planted;
A time to kill, and a time to heal; a time to break down and a
time to build up;
A time to weep, and a time to laugh; a time to mourn, and a
time to dance;
A time to cast away stones, and a time to gather stones together; a time to embrace, and a time to refrain from embracing;
A time to get, and a time to lose; a time to keep, and a time to
cast away;
A time to rend, and a time to sew; a time to keep silent, and a
time to speak;
A time to love, and a time to hate; a time of war, and a time of
peace (Eccl. 3:1-8 KJ).

WE MUST LEARN TO BASE THINGS ON WHO WE ARE, NOT ON WHAT WE CAN OR CAN'T DO.

Eventually we begin to let go of the memory of the person
we used to be, because we come gradually to accept that we
are never going to be that person again. We allow positive
things to begin to surface and come to light, and we dwell on
those things instead: the fact that we can still think and talk and
touch and GROW. And always, above all, that we still have
Jesus.

I struggled for so long to believe that He still loved me. I
struggled with *a lot* of unbelief . . . in healing, in a God who
really cared, in the fact that every hair on my head was numbered. But gently, slowly, the Holy Spirit wooed me back and I
began to look for a purpose in it all. I began to tread on higher
spiritual ground, because I was consciously taking my eyes off
myself and putting them on Jesus, and on *His* will, *His* timing,
His purpose, not mine.

But you will also begin to search again for Jehovah your God, and you shall find him when you search for him with all your hearts and souls. When those bitter days have come upon you in the latter times, you will finally return to the Lord your God and listen to what he tells you. For the Lord your God is merciful, he will not abandon you, nor destroy you, nor forget the promises that he made to your ancestors (Deut. 4:29-31, LB).

Lloyd Ahlem says that,

The key response to someone coming out of crisis is the spontaneous expression of hope. He is no longer wistfully hoping that someday life will get better, he is genuinely confident and making plans based upon this confidence.

Another key sign that reconstruction is going well is that reattachments are taking place. New persons are being chosen to replace lost ones. New jobs replace old ones. New homes become new places for roots to go down. New spiritual wells are dug for sating thirsting souls. . . . "The old things are passed away, behold, all things have become new" (II Cor. 5:17, KJ).

Along with reconstruction goes the need for reconciliation. This word has important meaning for the final phases of the sequence of coping. In normal human crises and changes, people around us get hurt. We are troublesome when we are in trouble. When we feel guilty we blame others. We are downright inconvenience and problem to others when our lives are in tough situations. When we enter the reconstruction phase, it's time for some reconciliation as well.[2]

The following poem came in the mail to me in a birthday card from a very dear friend:

Life – sweet life!
It's a celebration . . . a constant source of jubilation
Each sunrise, a gift
The dawn supplies afresh . . . new hope
If night, the thief has been,
For failing strength is much renewed

When blanketed in Slumber
And peace – filled dreams have often rescued minds
With care encumbered.
Rejoice with every breath – each thought.
Express your jubilation
And grab the vision,
See the truth – life is a celebration!
For even when you have no strength
And cannot carry on,
And must sit back in forced repose . . .
This does not stop the song!
It still resounds from tree to tree
Echoing life's sweet melody
It never ceases – there are just times we refuse to listen
It is our choice to hear life's song
Or turn a deafened ear
No matter what our limitations, there's always cause for Cele-
bration
So choose participation in the dance of life!

At the bottom of the poem was this note: "Happy birthday, dear friend. May it be just one day of a lifetime filled with blessings and the deep-rooted knowledge that He is all you need to have joy abundantly. Please don't think I take your situation lightly, for truly I don't. I only desire for you to rise above it and experience all our Lord has for you – in complete contentment and fulfillment. I love you dearly, Gaye."

I have to admit that when I first got this letter, I was crushed. I felt she was in essence saying that I wasn't doing a good enough job of coping or keeping my act together, and that I was refusing to "listen to life's song," as she put it. But then I thought about it alot for a couple of days, and came to realize that she was in fact, *encouraging* me – daring me to be all that I could, even though it seemed my life was over.

And that day was a turning point for me. My friend had wisely realized that it was time for my grieving period to come to a conclusion, and she was gently, lovingly inviting me to grow beyond it. And I did. That day I turned a corner. My flood of tears was over, and I never looked back.

ACCEPTANCE IN OUR ENVIRONMENT

When acknowledging the reality of illness, psychologist Franklin Shontz says,

> A person typically begins by hoping that each mastery of new situation will solve his problems once and for all. For example, a patient with paraplegia may begin to accept his condition by believing that once he is able to ambulate and drive a car, his struggle will be over. Experienced rehabilitation workers know that, in addition to the minor frustrations of learning necessary skills, increased mobility will create difficulties that were not foreseen. The patient may have to solve the financial problem of purchasing a specially equipped car. Because mobility means re-entering the institutional environment, he must learn to deal with staring and devaluating pity. He will find himself in an architectural environment that makes few allowances for persons in wheelchairs or on crutches, and in an economic environment in which hiring the handicapped is regarded as an act of charity.

We must keep in mind that our acceptance level may come at a different rate than that of our friends, spouse, children or employers. We may be an "embarrassment" to them in public. When I was still in a stage where I could not get around well on my own, I mentioned using a wheelchair to my husband. For a long time he would either change the subject or else abruptly change our plans to something that would not require walking. After watching this happen a number of times, I finally asked him point blank what the problem was. And incredibly, he told me that *he* would be too self-conscious to be seen with me in a wheelchair. I found this hard to swallow, since I felt that if *I* wouldn't be too self-conscious, why should he? By the same token, I was visiting friends in another city without my husband and we decided to go to a museum. "How about if I rent you one of these handy-dandy wheel chairs here at the desk?" my friend suggested without my even having to ask him. And he made a game of it, zooming me around that museum until I was afraid we were going to be thrown out for disturbing the peace. That was just one small difference in two different people's personalities, but what difference it made to me. And in the same way that we hope that people will accept us and our illness, we must accept them and their reactions to our illness.

If we keep the right perspective about our illness – that it's just our "cross" that we have to bear, and that everybody has one, it will help other people put it in the right perspective also. A sense of humor can't hurt, either.

I remember the day I decided to get out and get some fresh air with my husband and some friends. We were going to go to one of our old favorite hiking spots (I was quite a hiker in my day), but now I would just do as much as I could on a nice flat trail and sit down to rest frequently. As we were ready to leave the house, I went and got my trusty old hiking boots out of the closet and put them on. I laced them up, grabbed my coat, and started for the door. But I suddenly stopped short and just stood there, and I burst out laughing. My husband stared at me. "What's so funny?"

"Me," I answered. "I can't hike in these things. I can't even *move* in these things!" And my hiking boots, that were so well-loved and well-used, went back into the closet for good, because now the same legs that used to hike in them read their sturdy heaviness as cement blocks tied to my ankles.

One definition of the word *adventure* is "to venture oneself down a path unknown." We have been handed, through our illness or disability, an entirely different set of life's circumstances. We will go places we never would have gone, meet people we never would have met, done things we never would have done. With this new set of circumstances, we have the opportunity to become bitter . . . or better.

One man told his story:

> When I was seven, I was hit by a car, had my face crushed, and was pronounced clinically dead at the scene. By some miracle, I lived and am now 44.
>
> I was teased mercilessly in school for being ugly. Potential employers asked about my appearance. Even my wife blamed me for my poor reconstructive surgery. For years I was hurting. But then I learned that no opinion of me is more important than my own.
>
> I'm now a minister. Hardly anyone criticizes my appearance anymore because I accept myself. And I help others. I may have a physical deformity, but it's easier to accept than a deformed character in a beautiful body. God values us for what we are in our hearts.

Ivy Guntner was a New York high-fashion model with a lucrative career when she found out she had cancer. Four days later, they amputated her leg.

"I cried for a year," Ivy said during a recent talk show on television. This once slinky, sexy model, so used to making "entrances," said,

> I now had three choices: I could crutch in, wheel in, or God forbid, *crawl* into the bedroom while my husband waited. But we decided to look at this as a life adventure . . . because this was something we had to live with for the rest of our lives.
>
> I wanted to be normal so bad. I wanted to get back in front of the camera because I had been doing it for so long, it felt like home.

While Ivy was still in the hospital after her amputation, her agent came to see her to tell her that she was not going to renew her contract. "She provided me with my first challenge," Ivy said.

I had always wanted to work for Yves Saint Laurent, but he had his stable of girls that he used, and that was it. Well, I was bald now from the chemotherapy, and I knew he had models in Paris who were shaving their heads. So I went to his office, dropped my lucite cane at the door, and said, (pointing to her head) "How many other models in Atlanta would do this?" He hired me on the spot!

I will welcome happiness, for it enlarges my heart,
Yet I will endure sadness, for it opens my soul.
I will acknowledge rewards, for they are my due;
Yet I will welcome obstacles, for they are my challenge.

Og Mandiano

In a booklet put out by the National Multiple Sclerosis Society, there is a section titled "How Does One Learn to Live With MS?" We can substitute the name of any chronic illness or disability and it is still sound advice:

a) Concentrate on your abilities rather than your disabilities.
b) Take one day at a time. The nature of (a chronic illness) poses uncertainties about the future and it is more effective to direct your energy toward solving today's problems rather than worrying about tomorrow's.
c) Adjust your goals to realistic levels so that you will be able to reach them.
d) Enlarge your scope of values; attach importance to qualities other than physical prowess.
e) Measure your success by what it is possible for you to accomplish, rather than what others can accomplish.

f) While you should avoid dwelling on your problems, it is important to express your feelings and concerns to appropriate people – spouse, close friends, or a professional. Keeping them bottled up inside can lead to an "explosion" when they do come out.

g) Keep as active as you can within the limits imposed by (your illness). Limiting your activities does not mean withdrawing from the world and social contacts.

h) Be able to ask for and accept help when necessary: try not to demand it when you don't need it.

And last of all, and most important: Remember that you must accept yourself before you can expect others to accept you.

> I am only one, but I am one
> I cannot do everything,
> But I can do something.
> What I can do, I should do–
> And with the help of God,
> I will do!
>
> Everett Hale

"When a faithful person has accepted his illness, it is experienced as a restoration of a fellowship with God that seemed broken by the tragedy. God is experienced as near instead of absent; as a friend rather than an enemy; and as a daily guide rather than an enigma."[3]

Endnotes

1. Cox-Gedmark, J. *Coping With Physical Disability*, (The Westminster Press, 1980), p. 55.

2. Ahlem, p. 60-61.

3. Quote, John Baggett, Director of North Carolina Alliance for the Mentally Ill, and author of *When Mental Illness Strikes in a Family of Faith*.

4

THE SPIRITUAL BATTLE

Whatever is born of God overcomes the world; and this is the victory that has overcome the world – our faith (I John 5:4, NIV).

I spent a lot of time in spiritual limbo after I became ill. I never was able to bring myself to walk away from the Lord during all of my anger and fear and feelings of betrayal, but I just couldn't seem to bring myself to fully trust the Lord again, either.

Whereas, before I was always willing to pray out loud and share what the Lord was doing in my life, now I was mum. If someone brought up the Lord in conversation, I changed the subject. I couldn't relate to their joy or their growth. Maybe I was even coveting their easy, flowing relationship with the

Lord, untried and unbroken by the heartbreak and reality of a life-changing illness. I just simply withdrew, checked-out, sat back and waited. . . .

> I am still confident of this:
> I will see the goodness of the Lord
> in the land of the living.
> Wait for the Lord;
> Be strong and take heart
> and wait for the Lord (Psa. 27:13,14, NIV).

On the one hand, we have God, who has allowed this illness in our lives for a purpose: growth, maturing, strengthening, deepening our faith.

But on the other hand, we have Satan, just waiting for an opportunity to use this time of testing against us. He knows two things: 1) We're weak, and if he's crafty enough, he'll be able to steer us away from seeing this as from God and as a growth experience, and, 2) if he can get our eyes off God and onto the loss and pain, he has a good chance of getting us to walk away from the Lord entirely. Satan has a lot to gain here and *we have a lot at stake.* Our "lights" are in danger of being permanently snuffed out.

I personally can't think of anything Satan likes better than a defeated Christian. It doesn't matter whether Satan himself throws us a curve ball and we go down for the count, or the Lord sets up a test or trial and we fail it, either way we're defeated and Satan is immensely pleased.

> I want to remind you that your strength must come from the Lord's mighty power within you. Put on all of God's armor so that you will be able to stand against all the tricks and strategies of Satan. For we are not fighting against people made of flesh and blood, but against persons without bodies . . . so use every

piece of God's armor to resist the enemy whenever he attacks, and when it is all over, you will be standing up (Eph. 6:10-13, LB).

You are in a battle. The test (illness or disability) may be from God, but Satan is going to try to wrestle the glory from Him at every turn. And the only person who can keep this from happening is *you*, through your faith, trust and hope in a divine plan for your illness. As my pastor, Pastor Harley Allen, said in a sermon on suffering, we create *antagonism* in Satan as we move through this world, because we are children of God. Satan seeks to wreak havoc in our lives, our health, our marriages, our friendships, and our relationship with God. (BINGO. Chronic illness and disability cover every one of those areas from square one.) "God intended that the world would reflect His glory," said Pastor Allen. "Pain is the graffiti that Satan has scrawled across the face of God, His beautiful landscape, and God's people. It's Satan's way of defaming God's reputation. When was the last time that Satan was blamed for war, teenage pregnancy, or a drug overdose? But people always immediately say, 'Where was God in all this?' "[1]

> Be sober, be vigilant; because your adversary the devil, as a roaring lion walketh about, seeking whom he may devour (I Pet. 5:8, KJ).

Mario Murillo discusses attack from Satan in his book, *No More War Games:*

> After suffering a severe attack, many believers accuse God of failing or going back on His Word. But the failure lies in the fact that we have filtered scripture though our cultural preoccupation with escape.
> The needed information was there all the time. The Bible

teaches warfare. Triumph is promised, but *only* if we learn to fight the good fight! "Fight the good fight of faith, lay hold on eternal life, whereunto thou art also called, and hast professed a good profession before many witnesses" (I Tim. 6:12).

"Escape" is the key word here because Americans long to escape. We want to void effort, struggle, confrontation; in essence, we want to escape war.

We believe in the instant cure: the right pill, the appropriate button. Whereas character and greatness were once the product of the furnace of affliction, now we seek to microwave them into existence. It is a fantasy to want the benefits of effort without actually exerting effort and to want triumph without contending for it according to the rules.

America is finding out that escapism quickly reduces its victims to addicts without incentive. Life is an equal opportunity destroyer. Everyone will have a turn at a crisis that will reveal the substance of their foundation. Hollow anchors will fail, stage props will fall, and our false cures will explode when we need them most.[2]

"My faith in God is secure," you might be saying. "I would never walk away from the Lord, no matter how bad things got or what Satan did."

Good! But there is a difference between hanging onto our faith by a thread – and being a growing, productive Christian. A *big* difference. And this is what the Lord says we need to do:

Applying all diligence, in your faith supply moral excellence, and in your moral excellence, knowledge; and in your knowledge, self-control; and in your self-control, perseverance; and in your perseverance, godliness; and in your godliness, brotherly kindness; and in your brotherly kindness, Christian love. For if these qualities are yours *and are increasing, they render you neither useless nor unfruitful* in the true knowledge of our Lord Jesus Christ (II Pet. 1:5-8).

So let's run a quick check. Are we, because of our weak bodies, being rendered useless or unfruitful? Are we at a complete standstill in our faith? Satan doesn't care whether or not we're gaining ground, just so long as we're at a complete standstill, doing nothing – God's kingdom can't be furthered *that* way.

> WE KNOW THAT SATAN WANTS TO DESTROY.
> HE COMES TO STEAL, KILL, AND DESTROY.
> BUT JESUS CAME TO GIVE LIFE,
> AND GIVE IT MORE ABUNDANTLY

GOD'S PURPOSE IN TRIALS

LORD, HELP US TO REMEMBER
TO PRAY ABOUT OUR
ATTITUDES

Count it all pure joy, my brothers, whenever you face trials of many kinds, because you know that the testing of your faith develops perseverance. Perseverance must finish its work *so that you may be mature* and complete, not lacking anything. If any of you lacks wisdom, he should ask God, who gives generously to all without finding fault, and it will be given to him (James 1:1-4, NIV, emphasis mine).

God's goals for us are to be mature and Christ-like and to possess wisdom and knowledge.

Have you ever heard someone say, "Don't ever pray for patience, because God will give it to you?" God rarely hands us anything on a silver platter. Just like a wise earthly parent, He makes us work for things. The same holds true for maturity, wisdom, and knowledge. God's system for achieving these things in our lives is often trials. We all want these things

71

overnight, but God worked in Abraham's life for 25 years before He fulfilled His promise through Isaac, and 13 years in Joseph's life before he was allowed to become second in command to Egypt!

The English meaning of the word "patience" is very passive; the Greek says it better: Not simply to bear things, but to turn those things into something *great* in our lives. "When He hath tried me, I shall come forth as gold" (Job 23:10, KJ).

What is more precious than gold in this world? Testing is to refine us, to fit us to God's purpose and plan for our lives. It is to build up our spiritual muscles so that we can patiently endure what life throws at us. Think of how much more useful we are to the Lord when we are strong, rather than when our faith is frail and weak.

> Therefore, we do not lose heart. Though outwardly we are wasting away, yet inwardly we are being renewed day by day. For our light and momentary troubles are achieving for us an eternal glory that far outweighs them all. So we fix our eyes not on what is seen, but what is unseen is eternal (II Cor. 4:16-18, NIV).

And let us not forget that these "tents," our earthly packaging that makes us groan, are also temporary, and we will all be given brand new tents someday. Paul goes on to say in II Corinthians 5:1:

> Now we know that if the earthly tent we live in is destroyed, we have a building from God, an eternal house in heaven, not built by human hands. Meanwhile we groan, longing to be clothed with our heavenly dwelling. . . . Therefore we are always confident and know that as long as we are at home in the body we are away from the Lord. We live by faith, not by sight. . . . So we make it our goal to please Him, whether we are at home in the body or away from it. For we must all appear before the

judgement seat of Christ, that each may receive what is due him for the things done while in the body, whether good or bad.

Trials can: discipline us (Heb. 12:7-9), mature us (James 1:2-4), and refine our faith (I Pet. 1:5-7), but most of all, God can be glorified through them, as Jesus told His disciples about the man blind from birth: "Neither this man nor his parents sinned," said Jesus, "but this happened so that the work of God might be displayed in his life" (John 9:1-3, NIV).

DON'T FOCUS ON THE PROBLEM, FOCUS ON THE GOD WHO HAS ALLOWED THE PROBLEM TO MAKE US MORE LIKE HIM.

Kathy Perdue, the C.E.B.V. patient shares: "God knows best, and I had to accept that. Something good always comes of things like this. I look at this as a learning experience. God has the best for me in life, and it's out there for me to grab. This *is* for a purpose, because I have given Him my life to do with as He wishes."

THE ANSWER

I've spent hours and hours in prayer searching out the answer to the question "Why?" I could just not see a purpose in all of it. And then people would come up to me and say "Your faith has shamed me." Or, "Your faith has astounded me, cleansed me . . . and I know God is doing something special in and through you."

One day it just clicked. That was it! That was all there would ever be to the issue, I was just making something very pure and simple very complicated. The answer to all the questions was FAITH. The reason for my illness was to test my faith. The good that would come of my illness was the example of faith I could be for others, including unbelievers. I could touch lives, open eyes . . . it was all just a test. Was I passing or failing? Up until now I thought I had been failing miserably, because I had taken as my goal restored health. But that was a goal born of the world's system, not God's system. His goal is always to fashion us into the likeness of His son, Jesus. And Jesus' faith was tested at every turn of His life.

These trials are only to test your faith, to see whether or not it is strong and pure. It is being tested as fire tests gold and purifies it – and your faith is far more precious to God than mere gold; so if your faith remains strong after being tried in the test tube of fiery trials, it will bring much praise and glory and honor on the day of His return (I Pet. 1:71, LB).

GOD'S PURPOSE IN PAIN

WE MUST COME TO THE POINT WHERE WE CAN TELL GOD, "I WANT *YOU* MORE THAN I WANT AN ANSWER. I WANT *YOU* MORE THAN I WANT GUIDANCE."

In Twila Paris' song, *Do I Trust You, Lord?* she says, "I will trust You, Lord, when I'm blind with pain, You were God before, and You'll never change. . . ." The concept of being blind with pain is one that I don't think many Christians like to face, because we like to picture ourselves as *strong*. But I have been quite blinded by the pain of my illness –physical pain, emotional and mental pain – and I believe it was the *pain* that blinded me to God's love and caring through it all. I believe it was where the feeling of "separation" of God came from. It wasn't anything on His part, (though I felt sure it was), or anything on my part (I kept praying it wasn't), but instead that monster, PAIN. Which only makes sense, because who is the author of all pain and suffering? Satan. Satan is waging a battle here on earth, and although God will, through Jesus, eventually snatch the keys of hell and death from him in the final round, the battle is still raging. But as I heard an evangelist say one time, "Praise God, we know how the book ends!" We know who wins the war. It's like reading a novel like *Gone With The Wind*, or watching a movie about the civil war, and getting all engrossed in the South's battle. No matter how caught up in it we get, or how emotionally wrought, in the end we know who wins.

Right now we are totally caught up in the battle, and sometimes we just want to lay down our weapons and slink off home. But stay strong and be of good cheer, dear soldier – we know who wins the war!

God's grace is sufficient. "God's grace" literally means "God's help." Instead of kicking and screaming, "God, get me out of this thing!" we can say, "God, get me *through* this thing," because of His grace. In the face of hurt and pain, Christ offers grace, and He offers to let His glory shine through us. It doesn't make the pain any less painful, and it doesn't make the difficulty any less difficult, but it *does* fill the pain with strength and it fills the pain with purpose.[3]

> Since Christ suffered and underwent pain, you must have the same attitude He did, you must be ready to suffer, too. For remember, when your body suffers, sin loses its power, and you won't be spending the rest of your life chasing after evil desires, but will be anxious to do the will of God (I Pet. 4:1,2, LB).

For God sometimes uses sorrow in our lives to help turn us away from sin and seek eternal life. We should never regret his sending it (II Cor. 7:10, LB).

I am comforted by this truth, that when we suffer and die for Christ it only means that we will begin living with him in heaven. And if we think that our present service for him is hard, just remember that someday we are going to sit with him and rule with him. But if we give up when we suffer and turn against Christ, then he must turn against us. *Even when we are too weak to have any faith left*, he remains faithful to us and will help us, for he cannot disown us who are part of himself, and he will always carry out his promises to us (II Tim. 2:11, LB, emphasis mine).

I feel the need to insert a word here about coping with physical pain. While writing this book, I began one evening to feel my back and neck "cramping up" and I asked my husband to rub it. By time for bed the pain had greatly escalated, and I spent a sleepless night unable to turn over or turn my head without physically lifting it from the pillow with my hands. The next day I was no better, and the following day, even worse (I didn't think it was possible). The pain was excruciating and I was totally incapacitated. It felt like someone had hit me in the back of the head with a brick and I was nearly cross-eyed with pain. My husband said I was "cranky." All I wanted to do was lie in the middle of the floor and scream.

During this time my mother called and I told her that after a week of this, I wished my body would just get it out of its system and that it never had the audacity to do this to me again.

"Try having that for years," my mother said.

"I don't get it."

"Try having that kind of pain for years. That's what arthritis of the neck feels like."

My mom has had arthritis of the neck for many years and is

on permanent disability for it. She is on medication every day. But *this* kind of pain? I found it hard to believe. I wanted to say, "Mom, you *can't* be in this much pain. You rarely complain. You can't know what this is like!"

And then I caught myself. So this was the way people viewed my illness! "She *can't* be that tired. Her joints can't ache *that* badly." I was unconvinced that my mother could be in that kind of pain, though I love her dearly and believe every word she says. Why should mere acquaintances believe me?

My mother has anesthetized herself to her situation in all the same ways that I've anesthetized myself to mine. She went through anger, denial, etc. and finally came out on the other side at acceptance. She accepts her pain just as I accept my fatigue. My mother can run circles around me energy-wise. She attends an aerobics class three times a week that I couldn't begin to get through once. But amidst all this energy, there is unrelenting pain.

This episode with pain taught me many things. I found myself praying fervently that it would go away immediately, but more than that, that it would, please God, not be anything permanent, because I couldn't face pain like this every day for the rest of my life.

In essence, I was being thankful that I "only had C.E.B.V."; that I wasn't physically disabled by blinding, crippling pain. I could live with overwhelming exhaustion, aching joints, and feeling like I was dragging sand bags around with my body all the time, but please, not *this*. . . .

And then I understood what some of my sisters and brothers whom I was writing this for were really going through; a daily battle with grind-your-teeth-together, squeeze your eyes shut kind of pain. The kind that makes you want to crawl into a corner, curl up in a ball, and lie there and whimper.

And if that is where you are today, my friend, my heart breaks for you.

I pray that you have supportive people around you who will do for you physically what you can't do for yourself. I pray that you have at least one friend who will listen to you rant and rave and complain and rage against God and your situation, and then when you're done, will still be there when you start in all over again.

But mostly, I pray for a seed of understanding within yourself that you are a person of worth, even if you're totally incapacitated by pain. You still have a mind and spirit that can grow and feel and think and love and reach out to people and draw closer to God. Yes, it's all an effort. Yes, it seems grossly unfair.

And yes, God does still love you, just as He loved His Jesus as he hung dying and bleeding on a Cross. *We each have our crosses to bear.* For some of us, those are mental. For some, they are spiritual. (I think there's nothing sadder in this world than a Christian filled with doubt.) And for some of us, the cross is physical, a very real mammoth hunk of wood that we haul around with our tired bodies while it drives splinters into our hands.

Never fall into the trap of looking at the person next to you and envying them their health or freedom. Maybe their cross doesn't show on the outside, but they've got one. A mental or emotional scar from a past experience can leave a horror chamber embedded deeply in the mind and spirit of someone that never goes away. I have a dear friend who has lived with daily, unrelenting depression for years on end. No amount of counselling or medication has helped. Her life is a nightmare, and I find myself thanking God that my cross is only physical.

We should never offer to trade our pain for someone elses –

we might find out that we never knew the first thing about pain.

A LIFETIME OF SUFFERING

A sufferer once "raised a memorial" concerning a lifetime of suffering by writing the following thoughts on the matter:

> I am God's by right of creation, preservation, and redemption. Therefore He may do with me as He wills. To many creatures He sends health and strength; to me He has sent illness and pain from childhood. This I must accept as His gift, the gift of an all-loving, all powerful, all-wise Sovereign-Creator. "Shall the thing formed say to him that formed it, Why hast thou made me thus?" "As for God, His way is perfect."
>
> Second, I believe that I must accept pain not only as being *in* the will of God for my life, but as the will of God for my life. This is the background against which I must show forth His praise. Why this is so, I may not seek to know; I must accept it without question. More, I must know that His will for me is not only good and acceptable, but perfect. I must seek not only to accept it, but to embrace it, knowing therein lies my highest good.
>
> To this end I may not pray overmuch for the removal of pain, nor even for its cessation, but rather for the grace to bear it, the grace to benefit from it, and devotion to offer it up to God as a sacrifice of praise. I do not doubt for a moment that God is able to heal me absolutely in the flash of an instant; but He has not seen fit to reveal this as His will for me, and I must be content to leave the matter entirely in His hands. The scant strength I have for prayer must not be dissipated in seeking physical blessings, but rather be spent in seeking spiritual growth.
>
> Third, I believe that pain may be a way of knowing God. Through pain I may have fellowship with Jesus Christ, who, "though He were a Son, yet learned . . . obedience by the things which He suffered." Certain it is that the King of Glory is also the King of Pain, and that they who will reign with Him

must also suffer with Him. For most people this suffering is not of a physical nature; but is it not possible that for others it may be just that? "That I may know Him, and the power of His resurrection and the fellowship of His sufferings" must ever be the goal of every true follower of Christ. It may be presumptuous to suppose that one who is appointed to much physical pain can hope to know Jesus Christ in a special bond of the fellowship of suffering; but if pain is seized upon as an opportunity to know God in this way, I believe He will meet the seeker there. It is possible that such a one may come to know Him in a way that the completely well person perhaps can seldom, even never, experience or understand.

Fourth, I believe that pain may lead to a deeper prayer fellowship with God than may otherwise be easily experienced. When in the grip of severe pain, there is but one word my heart can utter, and that is the beloved Name, Jesus. For hours at a time I will wordlessly cry to Him, seeking only to stay my soul upon Him, too exhausted to make any request of Him; and at such times I know more complete communion with Him than at any other time in my prayer life. As George Macdonald puts it: "O God! I cried, and that was all. But what are the prayers of the whole universe but expansions of that one cry? It is not what God can give us, but God that we want . . . He who seeks the Father more than anything He can give is likely to have what he asks, for he is not likely to ask amiss."

Fifth, I believe that pain may provide a way of serving God. One of the hardest things to take about experiencing much physical pain is that it usually precludes much, if not all active Christian service. I wonder if pain itself may not be a source of service to God. True service is spiritual, consisting not so much in the doing as in the being; and the quality of service one may bring is not determined by its quantity, nor by much activity. If a soul that has been taught to suffer can look up into the face of the Savior and not only accept severe pain as from His hand, but thank Him for it, knowing that it is good, even perfect, just because it comes from Him, may not the soul be offering to God one of the purest forms of worship and service known to the spirit of man?

Finally, I believe that pain may be a training ground for future active and eternal service. "If in this life only we have hope in Christ, we are of all men most miserable" – this is especially true of the sufferer. The knowledge that pain forbids us much active Christian service in this sphere is one of its sharpest pangs. But this sphere is not all. Time is short, and Eternity is forever; and in that "last of life for which the first was made," "His servants shall serve Him." May not the sufferer who has known the sharp graving tool of pain in this life find he has been fitted for some special type of active future service for which no other preparation would have been adequate?

"To what purpose is this waste?" is the cry that is wrung from every human heart that must walk the way of pain. Physical suffering, with its accompanying disappointment, loneliness, loss, misunderstanding, and haunting fears, with its blighted hopes, its thwarting of earnest purpose, its wearing away of life in seeming uselessness –"To what purpose is this waste?"

In the perfect economy of God, there is no waste – unless I choose to deny Him the right to turn my pain into everlasting good.

I believe that in eternity, God's glorious fulfillment, His end, will more than justify His strange and difficult means; even the pain-filled life, if given back to him in love and trust, will be made to show forth the praise of the glory of His grace.

God keep me momentarily constant in this commitment and faithful to the totality of surrender that it demands![4]

THE HOLY SPIRIT'S ROLE

Remember, too, that when you can't pray (or think, or feel) anymore, that the Holy Spirit intercedes on your behalf.

The Holy Spirit helps us with our daily problems and with our praying. For we don't even know what we should pray for, nor how to pray as we should. But the Holy Spirit prays for us with such feeling that it cannot be expressed in words. And the Father who knows all hearts knows, of course, what the Spirit is saying as He pleads for us in harmony with God's own will (Rom. 8:26).

I have come to trust and depend on the Holy Spirit in His role. When I could not pray for myself with well thought-out phrases, I would feel my heart cry out in anguish, "I hurt. I'm scared. I feel betrayed. I need Your touch; I need to hear from heaven." These were just gut-wrenching expressions of a very needy soul, but eventually I came to understand that the Holy Spirit was filling in the gaps, smoothing out the rough edges, and carrying my urgent message on wings of love to the Lord.

The Holy Spirit is our comforter (John 14:15, 26). The role of the Spirit is as an intermediary between us and the Father when we feel separated from Him by sin or pain or hopelessness.

Trust Him. Rely on Him. Learn to lean on Him through the rough times. Let Him envelope you with the perfume of His love, sustain you, and give life-giving water to your parched lips. He will always be there for you.

Hold me for awhile, Jesus–
I think I need a good cry.
I've tried so very long to keep a stiff upper lip
And shield my fear with faith.
But right now I just need to cry for awhile.
Is that all right, Jesus?
Just hold me close and rock me,
And tell me about heaven.
Sing to me of your home of eternal rest
Where I can close my eyes gratefully
And sleep in blissful peace.
Hold me tightly, Jesus–
And chase away the anxiety.
Dry my tears with your robe of splendor
And shroud me in Your love.
Take my hand, dear Jesus–
And clasp it tightly

Wait here beside me until I fall asleep,
Until I've had my cry . . .
Please stay with me until Your Morning Light
Comes shining through once more.

Cynthia Moench

Endnotes

1. Allen, Harley, "Through the Fire of Suffering," Sept. 27, 1989.

2. Murillo, Mario, *No More War Games*, (Anthony Douglas Publishing, 1987).

3. Allen, Harley, from "Through the Fire of Suffering," a sermon preached Sept. 27, 1989.

4. Clarkson, Margaret, *Grace Grows Best in Winter*, (Wm. B. Eerdmans Publ. Co., 1985) pp. 59-62, citing "God's Purpose in Pain," from HIS magazine.

5

CHOOSING TO COPE

Karen Evans, a 33 year-old mother of two, has just been diagnosed with a degenerative type of arthritis that has a name a mile long that no one can pronounce. In essence, her hip-joints are disintegrating – ever so slowly. She is stiff and sore and in constant pain, so much that it often keeps her awake at night. She's begun to limp when she walks. So far the doctors have found nothing that significantly reduces the pain. She has been told, "Learn to live with it."

Watching her, I have been amazed. Quietly, faithfully, Karen has accepted her situation with wisdom and Christian maturity. Even with having to face the destructuring of her work environment and the financial ramifications involved, Karen has not given in to self-pity or the "Why me's?" She immediately shifted her focus to what she *could* accomplish, rather than what she couldn't. She is now working at home, having revived a latent talent for art, and is handpainting designs for a children's clothing company. To a psychologist, Karen would be known as a "good coper."

Mary (not her real name) is a well-known Christian author with Multiple Sclerosis. She has been a Christian since she was four years old and is now 30. When I interviewed her for this book, I was also amazed, but for other reasons. Mary has had MS for many years, but she is still angry about it. She is angry because her husband walked out on her because of her illness and left her with three children. "Don't tell me this is God's plan for my life!" she said flatly during the interview. "I don't want any pat answers. I can't believe that God really wants me in this position." She challenged my theology in this book that God does allow sickness in people's lives. Her vision of God seems to be a grandfather-type who only gives people exactly what they want, and she does *not* want to be a single mother with three children and MS. She seems to be looking at only the negative in her situation instead of searching for the positive. During our conversation, some things came out: an agent friend had called and offered all three of Mary's kids work in the movies. A marriage proposal had come from a man whom she was very attracted to, and whom she respected. She had been offered a job with a major Christian publishing house.

And yet, nothing good was happening in her life because the Lord was not doing what she wanted Him to – to take away her Multiple Sclerosis. We all need to ask ourselves if we are looking for direction from our situations and if the Lord wants some changes to result from them. Then we will be well on our way to being *good copers*.

The Chinese ideogram for *crisis* consists of two symbols: the figures that mean DEATH and OPPORTUNITY. If, when we begin restructuring our lives, we concentrate on the negative, stressful, fearful facets of our situation, we will become bitter, resentful people. If, on the other hand, we embrace the possibility for growth, we will be filled with hope and confidence.

THERE IS NO SUCH THING AS A PROBLEM WITHOUT A GIFT FOR US IN ITS HANDS.

Crisis has also been defined as the experience of "an acute situation where one's repertoire of coping responses is inadequate in effecting a resolution of the stress."[1]

"The intensity of [a] crisis is measured by the extent of *reorganization* required to cope with it."[2] If we do not adopt coping mechanisms and utilize them we will find ourselves under constant pressure and aggravation.

Much of it is a question of whether we *choose* to cope poorly or cope well. Says Kathy Perdue, the C.E.B.V. patient:

> Until you get your mental state in order, you have no coping skills. When I couldn't keep up around the house and the kids didn't help, I became infuriated and it was devastating. I had mood swings and depressions, but over a period of time I did learn how to cope with these. The main thing people need to learn is *their own* coping skills, to learn to approach it the best way they know how. If they don't have the necessary coping skills, they should *seek help.* And the most important coping skills are outlined in the Bible: to rely on God, and to keep our priorities straight.

OVERCOMING GUILT AND FEAR

Two areas that require great concentration of coping mechanisms are guilt and fear.

If given the chance, guilt is going to eat us alive, so we have to be on the lookout and ready to disarm it. If, when we became ill or disabled, we were isolated beings in a self-sufficient existence, guilt would not exist. But all of us are dependent in some way or another on someone else. We really do need each other. The problem arises when we begin to feel "needy" beyond what we can give in return. We feel guilty when we have to utter the words, "I need help."

We no longer feel in control and feelings of helplessness only compound the problem. Withdrawal and isolation usually follow. We figure that if we're not around people, then we can't be dependent on them. We begin to take total responsibility for our illness and the effect it has on other's lives, and this is where we can make a big mistake. We are *not* responsible. God made our bodies this way, so we can't feel guilty about what we can't do. It all rests on God's shoulders. When I realized that, I breathed a much-needed sigh of relief. God is in control. The minute we snatch that control back, life becomes murky. We take the weight of the whole world upon our shoulders. We feel *guilty*.

One basic reason for guilt as an ill Christian is because from the time we were little children we were taught that joy was achieved by putting things in this order:

Jesus

Others

Yourself

That's the only proper way for life to be lived. Now suddenly it seems that you (the bottom of the heap) have to be the main focus. *Your* body, *your* time, *your* energy – because that's what is essential now for you to take care of yourself. And that's very important. But the whole structure of life seems to be topsy-turvy and you're afraid of being branded selfish, egocentric, or a hypochondriac. Worse yet is having to admit that you're imperfect. Having to say "I can't," to a child or spouse can produce a lifetime of guilt in a society that tells us we must "Be all that we can be," "Go for the gusto," and "Have it all." The myth of "having it all" is hard on a healthy person; to the chronically ill, it is capital punishment.

That brings us to the issue of guilt and how it can affect our prayer life. At the onset of my illness I felt a barrier go up between myself and heaven – a closing of the trap door through which I caught glimpses of truth and comfort. This is the feeling I'm trying to convey when I say that I felt God was on vacation. The most shocking, devastating part of my illness was this separation from God, and I believe it came from a complete inability to pray for myself. I could move heaven for anyone else and their problems, but I could *not* pray for myself. I would sit down to open up my soul to God and I would cringe, shrinking away from having to utter the words, "I need help." I can look back at that time now and see that somehow it must have been related to guilt. It seemed selfish to pray for myself. I felt guilty for bringing God "my" needs. And maybe – just maybe, I felt guilty over unbelief. All my Christian friends were praying for me, petitioning God for me – He obviously didn't care, or wouldn't or couldn't hear their prayers. Maybe, deep deep in the corners of my heart, was I beginning to think it was all a hoax, that God had never existed in the first place?

Guilt, guilt, guilt for those thoughts and feelings nibbling at the corners of my mind! And of course I couldn't admit them to anyone. My feet were firmly planted. I was a rock. I never doubted, never cried, never hurt. Or so the world thought.

More guilt for not being honest about my feelings, for fear of destroying someone else's faith. I began to wear a mask and a bright, false smile. More guilt, more guilt!

I remember one day when a friend came up to me in the church foyer and said cheerfully, "So, how's Cyndi today?" And so weary of the game, I blurted, "Cyndi is feeling horrible today. I feel lousy and I'm tired of people telling me how good I look. And that's the truth." The complete shock on her face as she backed away guaranteed that I would never be honest about my feelings again. The mask went back on.

People don't *really* want us to be honest about our feelings and they don't really want to have to admit that we're sick, because then they are in effect admitting their own mortality. The less we say, the better they feel. And admitting we're sick is like admitting we have something wrong with us – a defect. But we need to admit it and get it over with, get it out in the open, and then people can begin to understand and help us.

I AM NOT RESPONSIBLE FOR THE WAY OTHER PEOPLE REACT TO MY ILLNESS AND I CAN'T CHANGE IT. I MUST BE MYSELF.

Lloyd Ahlem continues in *How to Cope With Conflict, Crisis and Change*:

> The beauty of the Christian experience is that because we have no masks to paste on, we have only God's forgiveness and peace to enjoy. We don't need to deny any feelings. God knows us better than we do, so there is nothing to hide. We may alarm our friends once in awhile, but no gut reaction is unknown to God. And He doesn't scare easily or fall off His throne with worry about how our experiences are going to turn out.
>
> Guilt can be a form of self-punishment. We decide that if people can visibly see how badly we feel for the havoc we're

wreaking in the their lives, then we will be forgiven for getting sick. But we can neither punish ourselves nor save ourselves. We need an act of belief based on the fact of a healing Savior to reconstruct our lives. When we bear the guilt of failure and have no one to give it to, we can be crushed.

A great truth is told in this regard in the Old Testament book of Job. Job was beset by calamitous events: loss of family members through death, loss of most of his assets through various disasters. As a result, a number of friends came to Job to comfort him. But they insisted that Job recognize his guilt as genuine. They decided that Job must be guilty of something because of the calamities that had befallen him. But Job would not yield to the temptation. He declared himself righteous.

The one who makes adequate adjustments in crisis has learned not to interpret his spiritual condition from either his emotions or events that come his way. Instead he identifies himself with the spiritual facts of life," says Ahlem, "That his righteousness is a gift that can be accepted without repayment. Any calamity that follows is not a refutation of his forgiven state. He can resist the temptation to feel guilt in either success or failure.

In the midst of feeling guilty and betrayed, we must learn to give the people who love us *credit*. We can become shortsighted and tunnel-visioned over our illness and begin to transfuse our emotions onto those we love, believing we know how they feel, when in fact we don't. Give them credit. They love us, they care for us. As humans they will obviously have an adjustment period, so we must give them this time. But then *believe* that they believe in you. I came to love my husband in a totally new light when I finally realized that he had been standing by my side, saying, "I believe in you. I trust you. If you say you're sick, then I know you're sick." He believed in me when it seemed no one else in the whole world did. But I couldn't see the beauty of this until I was finally ready to let go of my guilt.

Guilt is just another tool of Satan in this instance. He will try to rob us of our joy, build walls between us, and get our minds off God and onto ourselves. If we give into it, he is victorious, but this is a conscious decision on our parts.

FEAR

Psychologists refer to fear, guilt, anxiety, and hate as the critical emotions. They are most devastating to the personality if they persist. Furthermore, they are mutually reinforcing. if fear is allowed to persist in a time of crisis, it will tend to increase the possibility that the other critical emotions will take hold. If guilt is unresolved, it is likely that fear will continue longer than necessary. If fear and guilt persist, they will convert to anxiety, which will become a state of apprehension that will characterize the personality.[3]

I have experienced a lot of apprehension and fear in areas of my life that never existed before I became ill. I believe it has a lot to do with the "fight or flight" syndrome, a normal human reaction built into our defense mechanism for preservation of the species. But it is possible for it to get out of hand. The person seriously injured in a car accident may never feel totally comfortable riding in a car again. My mother was asleep in the car when she and my father were broadsided by a drunk driver thirty years ago. To this day she will not sleep in a car. When "bad" things happen to us in one area of our lives, the fear and apprehension can spill over into other areas.

My husband recently bought a ski boat. I had absolutely adored the water and skiing when I was a teenager. But the first few times out on the boat now, I was completely unable to relax, uptight, overwrought, a wreck! "What is the matter with you?" my husband complained. "Have you completely forgotten how to enjoy life?"

I had to thoroughly analyze my feelings and came to realize that because something as "bad" as my illness had been allowed into my life, I no longer felt in control of any situation. If one "bad" thing had happened, why not others? Why not a drowning accident? Why not a car accident? I felt constantly on my guard, and am still learning to deal with this.

Judith O'Brien, the Lupus patient, shared her fears with me: "I constantly go through the "what-ifs." What if I have to be put in a nursing home? What if I'm confined to a wheelchair? What if my spine continues to deteriorate and I become a vegetable? I don't want to be a burden to anyone."

My sense of loss of control went beyond my physical limitations and became embedded as fear in my life in general, my biggest fear being that of the future. It was a Catch-22, because on one hand I was trying so hard to trust the Lord, lean not on my own understanding, have faith and trust and hope. But my trust felt abused, because there was an unspoken trust in the Lord that I would not get sick in the first place. "So how," my poor pea brain screamed, "could I now trust Him with my future?" The future that would be so dark and bleak, for instance, if my husband died and left me a widow, unable to work and support myself because of my health. . . . My mind could supply endless scenarios – *if I let it.*

But I heard a very powerful yet simple statement of faith at a Barry McGuire concert one night. Barry is an amazingly grounded person, capable of conveying great truths very simply. And he simply asked, "How is God going to ever deliver us from our fears unless He puts us smack dab in the middle of them . . . then *delivers* us?"

That's scary in a way, isn't it? It snapped me back to reality like a short rubber band. The more I fear, the more God is going to have to test and try me to try to pry that fear out of my clutches. The more I hold onto my fear, the more vigorously God is going to have to scour my life of it. My, that sounds painful!

Being the broken down, imperfect being that I am, I can't claim that I'll ever have fear licked. But when I envision it as a curse – an unwanted disease in my life, I am better able to work at letting go of it . . . just turning my hands upside down and letting it fall out of my clutches, so that I can better trust the Lord. Because that's really the only way we can ever come before the Lord. Open-handed and palms-down.

Remember that bumper sticker which reads: "Nothing is going to happen to me today that God and I together can't handle"? My worst episodes with fear come when my mind conjures up the worst possible scenario and then I picture myself trying to live through it. But always, always my mind conveniently leaves God out of the picture. He is too great and good and kind and loving to be left out just so I can wallow in my misery.

> Do not fear, for I am with you, do not anxiously look about you, for I am your God. I will strengthen you, surely I will help you, surely I will uphold you with my righteous hand (Isa. 41:10, NASB).

> For God hath not given us a spirit of fear, but of power and of love, and of a sound mind (II Tim. 1:7, KJ).

> You will have courage because you will have hope. You will take your time and rest in safety. You will lie down unafraid and many will look to you for help (Job 11:18, 19, LB).

STRESS AND ITS EFFECT ON OUR BODIES

A chronically ill person may find himself trying to distinguish the crisis in his life as one of two things: either the actual *physical* complaints he experiences, or the reality of the process of having to completely *restructure his life.*[4]

It is important to look at the stress that living day to day with a chronic illness or disability can produce. Our society tends to view stress as an innocuous, subtle, by-product of today's world. But add to that "normal" stress a boat load of physical ailments, anxiety, fear for the future, financial difficulties and emotional upheaval, and it can add up to big problems.

Stress tends to accumulate over time, resulting in a stress spiral. When you are already stressed, a neutral event that you might not ordinarily respond to sends your stress level higher. With the next stress, you start out at a higher level, going even higher. Your chances of recovery from the stress arousal spiral diminish with each succeeding stress. Hans Selye, the "father" of the study of stress, feels that we all have a limited amount of adaptation energy to handle a stress. When your adaptation energy is gone, it's gone, and you break down physically, mentally, or both.[5]

Aesop knew this when he told us in his fable about the tree that survived the storm by bending instead of breaking in the wind. It's about "resilience."

Dr. Fredric Flach covers this in his book, *Resilience: Discovering a New Strength in Times of Stress* (Ballantine, 1989). He calls for an arsenal of personal qualities: self-esteem, independence, a sense of humor, discipline, compassion, an open mind, a religious base, and a network of a family and friends. When this resilience works, it leaves the person better equipped to deal with problems in the future.

"If people don't react and get insight from a crisis, then they have not adapted their style to be more effective," he says. "Instead of letting the problem hit them hard and then stepping back to assess the situation and make wise choices about how to rebuild or adapt, they try to shore up the status quo and preserve what they can. That can lead to a long-term, low-grade depression, which feeds mental and physical stress. The trick is trying to survive it, not control it."[6]

Stress can bring on a temporary flare-up of symptoms (known as exacerbations) in the phasic illnesses such as MS, Lupus, etc., as can other infections or excess fatigue. Keeping that in mind, we need to keep our environment as stress-free and running as smoothly as possible.

WHAT PATIENTS SUGGEST

One patient named Robert set about reducing the stress in his life, and finding out what made him happy. As a nurse, he had been working with dying children. After contracting C.E.B.V., he realized how stressful the job was, and eventually moved into administration. "I love it," he says.   Patients who have learned to reduce stress in their lives made the following suggestions:

1) Do what you really want in life.

2) Don't make the disease a life-style. Keep the focus on life, not on illness.

3) Find pleasant distractions.

4) If old activities must be curtailed, find ways to still enjoy them, such as playing in the water, rather than swimming.

5) When there's a choice, do the things that are most enjoyable.

6) Think positive about everything.

7) Make a dream list. Ideal job, salary, and work situation. Ideal home, location, neighborhood. Then find ways to come

as close as possible to these things.[7]

LEARNING LIMITATIONS

One of the most important areas that needs to be focused on, especially if you are newly diagnosed, is learning to set limitations for yourself. Many patients avoid this for a long time, thinking that it's a sign of weakness or a sign that they're "giving in" to the illness. "If I just run fast enough," a chronically ill person thinks, "then I won't have to admit that I can't keep up anymore." This in itself is a source of stress, because it means pushing our bodies beyond what they are able or willing to do now. And since stress needs to be avoided as much as possible, learning to listen to our bodies is the kindest thing we can do for ourselves. Many patients that I interviewed, especially those with phasic illnesses, have developed a plan of attack for dealing with life that is something like an "advance and retreat" plan for an army. Learning to prioritize is about *the* most important coping skill a patient can develop, I was told over and over. And that means learning to set priorities not only for today and tomorrow, but often a week or month in advance.

I like to picture my energy level as liquid in a one-cup glass measuring cup. The hardest thing is trying to guess *how much* liquid is in the cup each day, and how much I will choose to dole out for each project I assign myself. Some days I get up and the cup is about three-fourths full, and I can dole it out about one-fourth cup at a time. Those are my "good days." Then there are days when I get up and there's only about one-fourth cup in the entire measuring cup, and I must make difficult decisions about what to do and what to let go. The hardest part about this is when it directly affects someone else's life, such as when I've made plans with someone and then can't come through. The best way I have found to handle this is to be right up front with everyone in the beginning, and let them know that I might have to cancel at the last minute, and for them to please have an alternate plan in mind in case this does happen.

One patient says that she experienced a lot of relief when she finally realized that she didn't *have* to participate in every single thing her family did. "I finally came to a place where I could give myself permission to not go to the park that day, or not go swimming that day. If I pushed myself to go, I usually ended up tired and cranky anyway. This way, the kids had time alone with their dad, and I didn't have to feel like I was holding everyone back. We're all a lot happier in the end."

Karen Evans says that there are certain things she will give in to, but some of them she simply won't. She will take the needed time to rest now, often lying down in the middle of the afternoon. But she's not going to give up the ability to do things for herself any sooner than she has to. "We were talking about going to Marine World one afternoon, and I expressed doubt that I would be able to walk around that long. My kids got a big kick out of the idea of pushing me around in a wheelchair – it sounded like fun to them. But I refused. Some time the day might come when I'm going to *have* to be in one, and I'm not going to hurry that day along. If I give in to it now, I think I will only end up weaker."

"GOOD" STRESS

A concept that had never before entered my mind before I became ill was that of "good" stress. Stress is stress. It's anything that puts pressure on us. I was shocked when I realized that getting dressed up to go out wasn't much fun anymore because it took so much effort. By the time I got myself together, I was too pooped to party. The same with a weekend packed with social engagements – all fun things, right? Birthday parties, dinners, and trips to the mountains are wonderful diversions for someone with lots of energy. For someone chronically ill, these create what is known as "good" stress. Too many good activities will wear us out just like too many bad ones. The underlying pressure, though, is that while it's not too surprising to a healthy person that I might not want to spend a Saturday doing heavy gardening if I don't feel well, they can't understand why I wouldn't want to spend that same Saturday walking from one end of the mall to the other, "pleasure shopping." Few activities are pleasurable if you ache, are in pain, or are overwhelmingly tired. And this is where we have to learn to say "no" to good stress, just like we would to bad.

I'm not saying it's easy. It's especially hard for me to tell my husband, "No, I can't go camping anymore," or "No, I just can't fit three social activities into this weekend," when he is healthy and active and rarin' to go. We were always a "togetherness" couple – practically inseparable. We've had to learn to let go of that, and now he goes camping and fishing alone with a friend while I stay home and catch up on my reading.

What I have learned that has helped a lot is to plan ahead and see what's coming up on my calendar. If I have a big fun thing planned for the weekend, I will start on Wednesday or Thursday "saving up" my energy for it. I'll let scrubbing the bathroom go. I'll fix quick, easy meals and not let myself feel guilty over it. What I gain by letting certain things go is worth it to me in the end. I have learned that being a perfectionist is something only *I* demand of myself. I saw a cute saying one day that read, "Perfectionists are people who take great pains – and give them to someone else." And another one that I keep in mind is a refrigerator magnet which reads, "Dull women have immaculate houses."

If my illness has taught me nothing else, it *has* taught me what is important in my life. For each person, those things are different, but I have chosen to look at my illness as a way of getting to know myself and my Lord better. Illness "puts us between a rock and a hard place" and forces decisions on us that we might never have had to make before. Looking for the good and the "blessing" in this does not make us Pollyannas, but gives us a very real and effective coping tool to deal with the stress of our illness or disability.

RELIEVING STRESS

With chronic illness, our bodies are constantly stressed. But there is a way to relieve this stress, and that is through exercise. Now, before you groan and say, "I'm in too much pain!" or, "I'm too tired," please hear me out.

Stress by-products, wastes, and toxins build up in your system and can only be burned off by physical activity. It might take days for the wastes and toxins caused by a brief argument to be absorbed and flushed from your body without some physical action.[8]

Exercise is a tension releaser. I get frustrated because I can't jog or exercise in the same ways I used to, further adding to the tension! The key is *discipline* and although my whole body screams when I get down on the floor to exercise, I tell myself that I will feel better for it, and I always do. Bodily functions are regulated, my skin looks clearer, and I actually have more energy.

Swimming is an almost perfect form of exercise for someone who cannot support the weight of their own body for aerobic-type or even floor exercises. The water can buoy you up and give you a freedom you might never know again on dry land. Since many illnesses are often accompanied by a low-grade fever, the temperature of the water keeps the body from over-heating – which can cause added fatigue or dizziness. Many Y.M.C.A.'s now offer swimming classes for the handicapped, with instructors who would be there with the knowledge to help you if you should get into an emergency situation.

Another area that exercise benefits is depression. "Depression is an anti-movement condition," says Helena DeRosis, psychologist at New York University Medical School and the head of the self-help group Depressives Anonymous. "Depressed people can't move, they can't do, they're immobilized." The most natural anti-depressant is to get up and move your body. Almost any focused, physical activity can help battle depression. "Work every day," DeRosis says. "Take the biggest steps that seem possible. They don't have to seem easy, just possible."

When the body is in a state of rest, the blood moves more slowly, the poisons in the blood are not oxidized (cleansed away), and the system becomes sluggish.[9] Inactivity from lack of motivation, secondary to not feeling well physically, progressively inhibits the functioning of the part of the nervous system that automatically controls physical balance in the body.[10]

Dr. Marilyn Rubin, a professor of nursing at St. Louis University's School of Nursing, pointed out in an article in *The American Journal of Nursing* that while a night's rest in bed after a long, hard day usually leaves one feeling refreshed, forced bed rest caused by illness or injury can have the opposite effect.

Researchers have estimated that the functional losses after three weeks of total bed rest roughly equal 30 years of aging. While the effect of aging may be largely irreversible, the effects of bed rest can almost always be overcome. The major effects are related to the loss of gravity's pull on your body. As Rubin explained, when you stand upright, the body fights gravity in a "most helpful way." Your skeletal muscles contract, exerting pressure against veins and lymph vessels, which keeps fluid from pooling in your legs and feet. The anti-gravitational effort also makes muscle cells more robust and makes the bones stronger because muscle movement against gravity favors calcium deposition in your bones.

But when the mattress is holding you up, your skeletal muscles lose tone. "After just three days, a person on bed rest loses plasma and calcium, secretes less gastric juice, has less blood flowing through the calves and shows some impairment of glucose intolerance," wrote Rubin.

And so, you can see how very important it is to realize that our bodies are going through a special type of trauma during chronic illness and disability, not just our emotions.

We need to relax and take care of ourselves, but we also can't let ourselves slip into thinking that just because we don't feel good means we should crawl into bed and stay there. If so, we'll pay a very stiff penalty, physically, down the road for it.

MENTAL EXERCISE

It's also a high priority to keep our minds active and alert instead of just becoming t.v.-aholics or couch potatoes.

"Humans need a steady diet of novelty and challenge if we are to grow. It has only recently come to light that the *absence* of change – leading to boredom, passivity, or a sense of learned helplessness – can be stressful as an overload.

"Just as each of us seems to have an ideal body weight, our brains have an optimum level for input and change. When the level is too low, our brain signals us to seek out new experiences. When the flow is too great, the brain also has mechanisms to reduce the chaos and restore stability.

"Like a muscle, the brain grows and shrinks in response to everyday experience – the nerve cells actually become larger when stimulated, smaller when not. While scientists associate overstimulation of neurons with stress and other deleterious effects, it appears that too little stimulation can also cause the nervous system to go awry."[11]

Have you ever been home sick in bed and had a friend stop by? It took your mind off the pain in your body, and you no doubt felt better for awhile. But then after the friend left, you went back to concentrating on your body. Outside stimulation is terrifically important.

It's highly probable that chronic illness or disability will produce a preoccupation with "self," because the self is what we carry around in this body that has betrayed us and left us weak and in pain. To counteract this, we have to focus *outside* self.

Read, force yourself to take a class – even though it may not be a picnic getting there, or even sitting through it. But you might find that if you're placing your attention on what is being taught, your attention will not be on your weakness or pain.

Working with one's hands is a great tension-reliever, if you're physically able. When the hands are busy, the heart and mind seem to be given a freer rein to wander and relax and stretch and grow. Stimulate yourself to grow with a pottery or ceramics class, flower arranging class, weaving class, soapstone carving or woodworking class (work benches can be built wheelchair height also.)

Recently I took a four-hour paper-marbling class one dreary Saturday afternoon. (Paper marbling is an ancient art that you probably picture on the templates of old books.) Yes, I had to talk myself into going. Yes, I got very tired and had to go outside partway through class and recline the car seat to rest. (Most classes offer a lunch break, fortunately.) But I came away from the class with eight samples that I made with my own two hands – instant gratification!– that could be used as beautiful stationery to write my friends. My mind had been expanded and I no longer had to look at those beautiful designs and wonder, how in the world do they do that? Try something new!

If you're up to it, try to think of someone to visit who is possibly in even worse shape than you. You'll count your blessings.

PEOPLE ARE LONELY BECAUSE THEY BUILD WALLS INSTEAD OF BRIDGES.

Endnotes

1. Miller, K.S., and I. Iscoe, *The Concept of Crisis: Current Status and Mental Health Implications,* "Human Organizations," 22, (1963) pp. 195-201.

2. Shontz, p. 156

3. Ahlem, p. 48, 151

4. Ahlem, p. 86

5. Shontz, p. 157

6. Lewis, p. 100, 101

7. Daily Ledger-Post Dispatch, 23 July, 1989

8. Lewis, p. 105

9. Lewis, p. 37

10. Jackson, E.N., *The Many Faces of Grief,* (The Parthenon Press, 1977), p. 74.

11. Ornstein, Robert, Phd., and David Sobel, M.D., "Can You Psyche Yourself into Good Health?" *Glamour,* August, 1987, from the book *The Healing Brain,* (Simon and Schuster, 1987).

COPING IN RELATIONSHIPS

"EXPECT TO INVEST A GREAT DEAL OF TIME
AND ENERGY IN YOUR RELATIONSHIPS.
RELATIONSHIPS DON'T JUST HAPPEN,
THEY ARE CREATED."
                                    Leo Buscaglia

To My Family and Friends

I'm sorry.
I know you remember the me
That I used to be.
But that is not the me I am now.
There's nothing I can do about it,
And neither can you.
I know you feel shaken, worried,

And perhaps betrayed
Maybe you feel I've let you down . . .
But believe me, so do I.
Please know that I am doing the very best I can
To readjust myself to a whole new set
Of life's circumstances
And I pray that you'll try to adjust also.
Please don't forget
That if you can be there for me right now
(For however long "right now" is)
I'll try to learn to be there for you again someday.
Because, we really are all in this thing together. . . .

C.M.

Just as our perception of ourselves changes when we become chronically ill, so also do other people's perceptions change, and we need to understand and be ready for this. We have all seen a child point to a visibly disabled person and begin to ask questions, only to have the mother scold the child or drag him on their way. Children are innocently curious and open about disability. Adults are curious, but unless very rude, they usually try to hide it. But that does not stop them from having very definite thoughts and feelings toward the sick or disabled.

In *The Psychological Aspects of Physical Illness and Disability*, Dr. Shontz tells us:

> American culture has strong beliefs about proper behavior in response to pain. Ostentatious displays of suffering are regarded as evidence of character weakness, whereas the ability to endure extreme situations without outward signs of despair is admired as evidence of courage and personal strength. . . . The person who breaks a wrist "has a right to" a certain amount of

pain . . . the moral character of the sufferer is judged by the amount of distress he has a right to feel and the intensity of his display of discomfort. If he displays less suffering than he "has a right to," he is a hero. If he displays too much suffering, he is a cry-baby or a complainer.[1]

Ruth B. Purtillo, a registered nurse, said in an article in *Physical Therapy*:

The first few weeks following a person's accident or illness are attended by flowers, cards, numerous visitors, and constant encouragement. But the able-bodied grow weary. Their responsibilities are many and varied. They are disillusioned by the afflicted person's inability to return to the real world of involvement, independence, and responsibility. Sometimes they are even angry that the afflicted person "refuses" to come back home where he or she "belongs," or return to the job in order to lighten the work load. Then, just about the time the chronically ill or disabled person comes to full grips with the stunning reality of permanent impairment, the room is bare, the phone is silent, and the flowers have long since wilted.[2]

This tapering off of supportive relationships often is the most difficult reality the patient has to face in a chronic illness. On the other hand, a positive result of this process is that friends and relatives who do not disappear out of neglect, exhaustion, or despair often become more dear. This period is a time of testing the quality of relationships and discovering one's true friends.[3]

"NEVER TRUST A FRIEND WHO DESERTS YOU AT A PINCH"
Aesop

When I became chronically ill, I discovered who really cared about me, and who was in the relationship just for what they could get out of it. I found out who was willing to part with hard-earned cash. "Here," our friends Karen and Lamont said to my husband Jim, when we were going under with medical bills and I was at my mother's house being cared for 2,000 miles away. "Take this money and buy yourself a plane ticket to go see Cyndi." When Jim told me that on the phone so far away, I cried and cried. They were our "quiet" friends – they never said much, and I guess I'd never known how much they really cared about us, but now I did. And I will never forget their offer.

Sometimes the ones we thought we knew best turn out to care the least. There was the friend who, when I finally got a doctor to admit there was something wrong with me, exclaimed, "Thank goodness! Now I can go to the club and tell them all you're not a hypochondriac after all!" Talk about kicking someone while they're down.

Sitting out under a peaceful sky in lawn chairs one day, an old friend from far away (who had called up and invited herself and her whole family to come stay for the weekend) casually mentioned "how hard it had become to be around me," and how my illness now "colored our whole friendship." "I guess I'm just not good around sick people," she said. This came *after* I had rearranged my schedule, run to the grocery store, and cooked and cleaned for them the whole weekend. It wasn't as if I had been lying in bed or on the couch the whole weekend complaining. Her children had even asked my husband why they had to sleep on the floor instead of in *our* bed! I decided to save her the trauma of "coloring our friendship" any more.

I could go on and on, but you get the picture. You probably have a number of horror stories you could relate yourself. The sands of fortune shift and along with them shift every relationship in our lives, some for the better. Some disappear. I have made friends in the last few years with a number of chronically ill women. We get along well because we understand each other; there is a bond there that a healthy person cannot begin to form with me. We feel we can complain a little once in a while and know the other person *really* understands.

> ## "FRIENDSHIP BRIDGES THE GAP BETWEEN WHAT THINGS ARE AND WHAT THEY COULD BE."
> Roger Holmes

The friends who do stick by us can become a lifeline of hope in times we need it most, and we need to take care to treasure them. They are the ones who are willing to look beyond our illness or disability and see us for what we really are. Consider the words of Margery Williams' book, *The Velveteen Rabbit* (New York: Avon Books, 1975):

> "It doesn't happen all at once," said the Skin Horse. "You become. It takes a long time. That's why it doesn't happen to people who break easily, or have sharp edges, or have to be carefully kept. Generally, by the time you are Real, most of your hair has been loved off, and your eyes drop out and you get loose in the joints and very shabby. But these things don't matter at all, because once you are Real, you can't be ugly, except to people who don't understand."

At times, I have thought that it might be emotionally easier to have a glaring disability because people would see it, make a snap judgement of whether to accept me or reject me, and we could get on with the business of living.

As it is, I never know how much to say. Meeting new people is a wild guessing game. Do I *pretend* like I'm not sick, so the evening can progress smoothly? (All chronically ill people deserve Oscars for their acting.) Do I mention it casually, hoping to put myself on equal footing with them, and then have them plague me with questions all evening? Or do I just make a grand speech and get it over with, at which time the new person instantly sizes me up as a hypochondriac, because after all, who talks about their health at the first meeting?

Then there is not even knowing how much to say to the people who *know* I'm ill. Do I gently remind them that I'm sick? When I don't, they tend to think I'm "showing improvement," or else they expect too much of me. They wonder why I haven't had the chance to get out and find them a birthday present, when in fact, trudging from store to store, looking for just the right present is one of the hardest things I do.

It takes a lot of patience and determination for a healthy person to learn to listen, *really* listen to what we're telling them. They have to become private detectives, picking up clues and searching our eyes and body language for the real story of what's going on with us. It's much easier for them to gloss over the truth and play "let's pretend it's not there, and maybe it will go away." If they flatly ignore what we tell them or only listen superficially, it can only lead to trouble. Sometimes even when we speak plainly and spell out the situation, they only listen with "half an ear."

Early on in my illness, a couple invited us to make a trip with them. They lived six hours away, and they said we could drive to their house, spend the night, and leave the next day. They said they had borrowed a van so I would be more comfortable, and I could even lie down if I needed to. Great, I thought, they are really taking my illness into account, maybe I really can pull this off. I wrote and told them how slowly I moved, and that I have to stop and rest frequently. I told them I needed lots of sleep and I could not get an early start. I told them that the six hours alone to their house was a major undertaking. And it was. It was my first attempt at a trip and it went much worse than I expected. I felt nauseated the whole way, and when we finally arrived, I was exhausted and looking forward to a good night's sleep.

Then it happened. Our friends proceeded to give us the "schedule": We would be leaving at 6:00 A.M. the next morning. We'd have to rush the trip because he had to get back for an important meeting, etc., etc. I just sat there with my mouth hanging open, feeling hurt and confused. Hadn't they listened to *anything* I had told them? As it turned out, they went on without us, because there was no way I could have tackled that trip the way they were planning it. And it was all because they had heard me, but they hadn't really *listened*.

Sometimes people don't listen because they don't want to understand. Sometimes they simply *can't* understand. I missed a very important funeral in the life of our family because I was not at a point where I could handle a 12-hour car trip, and we could not afford the air fare because of all the medical expenses. All of the elderly folks in the family made it to that funeral, wondering why I wasn't there, when I was only "tired." They could not begin to understand, and I could not begin to explain it to them all. But feelings were hurt, I know.

There are some members of my family who I don't believe have fully accepted my illness even after five years. There's also an "order of responsibility" that is usually followed in families, and one sick member can throw that order entirely out of whack. I don't think my grandparents have ever fully understood that I now act like them, need care like them, dropped off at the door like them. They perhaps resent my "shirking my responsibility" as they see it, because I am not over washing their windows, but now need someone to wash mine. After caring for me through childhood, they came to expect that I would care for them in return, and now am unable. Chronic illness destroys life not only as we knew it, but also as we expected it to be.

WHAT DO I TELL MY CHILDREN?

In a booklet put out by the National Multiple Sclerosis Society, this question is discussed. Here is what they recommend:

> Depending on their age and maturity, children have varying needs for information and can absorb different amounts. They are quite perceptive and quickly sense when things are wrong.
>
> While they may not need to have the problem identified by name, they do need to be reassured, at some level, that their ill parent will not die and leave them alone. They also need to know that even if their parent must take a less active part in physical activities, and even though his or her role in the house may undergo a change, he or she is still able to provide the love expected of a parent.
>
> (Illness) is a family problem and children can be helpful as long as they are not overburdened beyond their years.[4]

Participate in activities with your children as much as possible. Your attention and presence are what they crave most – not your physical ability. Go to that little league game and cheer from your wheelchair. Have a favorite uncle or male friend teach your son to pitch while you give suggestions on technique.

And think creatively about areas that you can easily handle. One of my husband's favorite childhood memories is that his mother used to sit down and play rummy with him when he got home from school in the afternoon. There are always puzzles, chess games, or just sitting and listening to your child practice the piano. These are all ways to participate without a lot of physical exertion. The important thing is that you will be creating memories for your child of what you *could* do, not what you couldn't.

WHAT ABOUT MY SPOUSE?

Let's face it: chronic illness and disability have the propensity for wreaking havoc in our marriages, creating heartbreak and stress and misunderstandings.

The national divorce rate is now close to one in two marriages. In the marriages of the ill and disabled people I have interviewed, roughly the same statistics have applied. Perhaps it was easier for a spouse to say, "I'm leaving because of your illness," but there is a good chance that same spouse would have found a different excuse, also.

It's difficult to make any generalizations about handling this area in chronic illness, because each and every marriage is different. There's a good chance that if it was a solid marriage before the illness or disability struck, it will continue to be a solid marriage after. I'm of the school of thought that people either go into the marriage determined to make it last, or they don't. The only statistic I have to back this up is the fact that back when divorce was viewed with much more disdain, it happened much less frequently. Now it is almost fashionable for people to get out of a marriage to go "find themselves." If a spouse with a chronic illness provides them with the incentive to leave, they didn't need much incentive.

I have to admit that I worried a lot that my husband would leave me when I became ill. Who needs all this added stress? I thought. If he was given a choice between a sickly wife and a healthy one, why *wouldn't* he choose a healthy one?

I finally confronted him with my worries. He just looked at me incredulously. "I married you for better or worse," he said. "In sickness and in health, remember? They didn't just throw that in there because it sounded nice. . . .I have a vow to keep that I made before the Lord. What if it were *me* that had gotten sick. Would *you* leave?"

And then I saw how ridiculous my thoughts had been. Of course I wouldn't leave if he got sick. I would work even harder to love him and reassure him and protect him. And that's exactly what he's done for me.

I saw that the fear of his leaving was working against me just as fear in general in the other areas of my life had done. I had to turn loose of that fear – just let it go, and give it to the Lord, because otherwise it could destroy me. If I should lose everything, the Lord would still have to be Number One.

It is easier to turn things loose in life and "let them go" if we feel we at least have some measure of control over them. One area that bothered me a lot was the thought of what I would do if something happened to my husband and I was left alone to try to fend for myself in this world, unable to hold down a job. I stewed about this for a long time, also, but then I realized that it was at least something we could have some control over. The answer for us was insurance. A lot of people told us not to put our money into something like life insurance. It was much better to put that money into something like a C.D., we were told. But then we realized that what works for one person doesn't necessarily hold true for everyone. Life insurance would provide for me some peace of mind in the event of my husband's death. We bought enough to see that the house would be paid off and I would still have something left to live on. We also bought accidental death insurance, something that is relatively cheap for the coverage you get. These are things we never would have done had I not gotten sick. But drastic life circumstances often call for drastic measures, and we did what felt right for us in our own situation. If I were well, that money would have gone elsewhere. Everyone makes choices in life. Some people choose to have elaborate vacations, yet live in humble dwellings. Others choose to have lavish homes, yet can never afford a vacation. Try looking at your life in terms of what is right for you, not someone else, or some other couple.

If you have a spouse who has stood by you through this most trying time, thank God for him or her daily. If you are newly diagnosed and are both still adjusting, try to look at it as any other adjustment in marriage. If, when a couple had a baby and the baby was "difficult" because of colic or some other disorder, would they say, "That's it, we've had it. We're putting the baby out with the rest of the garbage for the trash men on Thursday . . ."? No way. First of all, it's illegal. Second of all, they would probably realize that it was just a part of life, an "adjustment period" they had to get through. Time marches on. Life changes.

The problem with marriages is that it *is* perfectly legal to put them out with the trash on Thursdays, and people do it all the time. So a couple needs to come to grips with the reality of the need to restructure their lives together, to decide what is most important to them, to decide that *their marriage* is important to them, and to do what is necessary to preserve it.

The same coping techniques apply here that have been outlined in the other sections of this book. The lines of communication must be opened up and each spouse must feel free to speak his needs. Needs change, and "thinking" that we know what the other person wants or needs is not the same as knowing. As a chronically ill person, you are not the same person your spouse married, and he or she needs to be told that, and *what* has changed. And you have to give your spouse the right to mourn his or her former life, also. Being the spouse of a chronically ill person, a "caregiver," is not what they foresaw in their future when they married you, but that is what life has handed them, and they need time to get used to the idea. Sometimes "time" really is the only thing that can heal a wound.

Says one couple: "We face whatever has to be faced, we just don't do it ahead of time. We have really learned to take it one day at a time."

Giving each other the right to his or her own life is very important now, because as one ill person and one healthy person, your lives are no longer the same. Try to let your spouse go. As a line from a song says, "Don't be afraid if I fly . . . a bird in a cage will forget how to sing. If you love me, give me wings. . . ."

Says one patient: "I made up my mind that I was going to let my husband go and grow, and be and become. If he decided to let me come along, I would go. And I have."

Learn to tell your spouse *exactly* what you are feeling. If you're having a "bad" day, say so, but try not to complain if it isn't necessary. Saying, "My legs feel like jelly today," lets your partner know what to expect from you that day, and keeps you from becoming irritable and resentful because he or she doesn't understand.

Talk also, about a different "master plan" now that you're ill. Your future together as man and wife will change now that you're ill. Give it time to see what changes in goals your health brings, then plan accordingly. Your future doesn't have to be worse: just "different." Just as in other areas of your life, now that you're ill, you have been given a chance to step back and see what is really important to you in life. My husband and I have found out how important "Play" is in life since I became ill. The added stress of the illness needs to be relieved, and playing was something that we'd never taken enough time for before. Now we do.

Endnotes

1. Shontz, p. 82-83.
2. Purtillo, Ruth B., MTS, "Similarities in Patient Response to Chronic and Terminal Illness," *Physical Therapy*, Vol.. 56, No. 3, (Mar. 1976): 280.
3. Chyatte, Samuel, M.D., p. 10.
4. Wasserman, Lynn, "Living With Multiple Sclerosis, A Practical Guide," (National Multiple Sclerosis Society, 1978) p. 15.

7

PRACTICAL DAILY APPLICATIONS

And then it came down to not how clean my house was, or whether or not I got the laundry done, but what kind of person I was, and what my relationship with the Lord was, really.

A patient

To say, "You need to restructure your life emotionally, mentally, spiritually and physically," sounds like a huge, almost unmanageable undertaking, I know, especially for someone who has little energy to begin with.

So the key has to be to start small, with little tiny steps, just as when a baby is first learning to walk. If we place too many demands on ourselves, we will become overwhelmed and feel like we have no control over our lives at all.

It helps to begin to re-think your lifestyle, down to the smallest detail. Even the most routine things in life can become major, intimidating hurdles when we are sick or disabled. The following are a few practical tips that I have found helpful, and I hope you will, too:

Set *little* goals for yourself. There was a time that I could do everything that I put my mind to, and still only needed six hours of sleep at night. Now I might do the laundry, or write a letter, or empty the dishwasher, and I have achieved my goal.

You may need to re-think your living situation. Do you *really* need this big house? This big yard? Should you keep a house with stairs that make you feel worse, or that you can't climb at all? Should you live so far out in the country that everything is a major drive? Or maybe it's the reverse – and you live in such a congested, noisy, busy area that you feel you never can relax. Make changes. What about a warmer climate? (I found warmer makes me feel better.) You have to become almost selfish in that you have to structure your life according to what's best for you. One thing I found that helped tremendously was installing a jacuzzi. It has been the best thing for my aching joints and tired muscles.

Rearrange your kitchen. Lower the cabinets. Lower your workbench to wheelchair-height. Put your washer and dryer up on a platform so you don't have to bend so far. Or buy a stackable set. I got a new refrigerator with the freezer on the *bottom* because I was always bending over to get into the fridge. I get into the freezer much less frequently. The freezer also has a pull-out drawer in it, so things don't slide all over the freezer like they used to.

After I got sick, I found going to the grocery store to be a highly exhausting expedition. I would drag myself up one aisle and down the next with only a vague idea of what I was going to serve that week. Now, I sit down for 30 minutes and plan out a menu of ten meals, right down to the desserts, look up all the recipes, note the ingredients, and troop off to the store. My husband started going with me to carry the bags, also. He doesn't mind, because this way he gets extra goodies into the house that I wouldn't normally buy. Now he doesn't stand in front of the cupboard anymore moaning, "There's nothing to eat in this house!"

One woman I heard about does her grocery shopping every two weeks also, but she is confined to a wheelchair. She moves a shopping cart to the end of an aisle, then proceeds up that aisle, placing the groceries on her lap. At the end of the aisle, she stacks them in the cart, then pushes the cart over to the next aisle. A stock-boy loads the groceries into the car for her, and she times it so that her husband will soon be home to unload them for her. (If you live alone, a neighbor could do this.)

Consider installing hand-controls to be able to drive a car. The Department of Vocational Rehabilitation will pay for hand-controls if they facilitate a return to the workplace. One man in a wheelchair bought a station wagon with the chrome luggage rack all along the top. He puts his wheelchair into the back of the wagon, and then grips the luggage rack to inch himself along the car to the front seat.

The President's Committee on Employment for the Handicapped, Washington, D.C., 20210 has put out the booklet, "Highway Rest Areas for Handicapped Travellers," and also a list of Guidebooks for Handicapped Travelers. You can also request guidebooks for handicapped visitors from the cities and addresses listed.

More than sixty Amtrak stations have been built or renovated to aid the handicapped. Amtrak will arrange your seating and sleeping accommodations to best serve you if you call their toll-free information and reservations line, 1-800-555-1212. Just ask for this information for "Amtrak."

Airlines will give you preferential treatment and put you on the plane first if you request it. Most airports have special carts with drivers that you can request to meet you if you prefer not to use a wheelchair and you can't walk far.

One Lupus patient says that people will come up and point-blank ask him what he has been drinking, as he stumbles along. He has solved this problem by using a cane. A patient may shrink in horror at the thought of using one, but a cane tells the world to watch out for you – and that you may need assistance. People may not understand the unsteady gait of a person with MS, Lupus, or C.E.B.V., but they do understand a cane.

A conventional tub or shower stall poses problems for a person who is too weak to stand in a shower or climb into a tub. Try placing a chair or stool in the tub and using a hand-held shower. If you are weak when you first get out of bed (as I am), try having a cup of tea or eating breakfast to give yourself time to get your balance before climbing into the shower. Be aware that legs often stiffen in sleep and that many times patients fall getting out of bed. If you feel a fall coming, don't try to brace yourself - you'll no doubt break something. Try to relax and fall like a drunk would.

Decide what your priorities are around the house. If having a super-clean house is important to you, hire a cleaning lady or a teenager to come in after school. On the other hand, if no one is all that fussy about meals, take the easy route out. No one ever died of malnutrition from living on hot dogs and macaroni and cheese. Go out to eat when you want a "nice" meal.

One woman cooks all day when she's having a particularly "good" day, and then freezes the meals for later. Casseroles freeze particularly well. I always bake double batches of brownies, cookies, etc. when I do it. I figure if I'm going to bother making a mess in the kitchen, I might as well do it big and get it over with. Everything goes into the freezer. Sometimes I cook double meals if I know I want to go do something "fun" the next day, and I won't have the energy to cook when I get home. Crock pots are life-savers for this reason, too. It all goes into one pot and then I can forget about it that day. The only trick is remembering to thaw something the night before.

Develop problem-solving skills. Identify the problem so it is clear in your mind, then write it down. Then list the pros and cons of your options. Now, choose a plan, and list the ways available to you to carry it out. Finally, ACT. There is nothing more paralyzing than not being able to make a decision. Chronically ill people who find themselves removed from the workplace often feel out of kilter with the world around them, and often it is because they now have too *many* options available to them. A workplace structure feels very secure. Total freedom can be intimidating. Focus on one goal at a time. Don't try to be Superman or Superwoman. Learning to pace yourself means stopping *before* you are tired.

Public Libraries have application forms for the service of free talking books through the Library of Congress, a boon not only to those whose vision is impaired, but those who find even holding a book up a struggle. Or consider large print books if your vision is impaired, such as is the case with many MS patients. Many libraries are beginning to carry a good cross-section of large print books.

Hospitals are beginning to offer classes to instruct patients and their families in ways to learn to live with a new disease or disability. In our area there are classes for diabetics, Lupus patients, those who have had colostomies, etc. Often times social workers or family therapists offer group counselling sessions for patients and their relatives to discuss their problems and fears and learn how others have coped.

Don't be embarrassed about asking for help. That was one of the hardest things for me to do, and yet I learned a little secret that has gotten me through it. Are you ready? *People like to help.* It makes them feel good to know they are doing a good turn. People *need* to feel needed. You may actually be cheating someone out of a blessing by denying them the right to help you. So ask. Let it be known around your church that you could use a little help trimming those bushes or mowing that yard. Or maybe your hands are too unsteady to do the mending anymore, there might be a mother whose children have all left the nest who is just looking for something to occupy her time.

My friends who are chronically ill and I often discuss the need to look at the options that *are* still available to us is life, rather than the ones that aren't. If we spend time thinking about the things that "got away" because of our illness or disability, we will continually be living in the past. We need to concentrate on our ability, not our disability.

These are just a few hints that have worked for me, and the list is not meant to be inclusive, but rather to get your mind rolling in the right direction. Sometimes we all need to learn to think in "new" ways . . . to unlearn or re-learn patterns, to start new traditions. It's all part of the growth process in this thing called life. We can either thrive on challenges, or we run from them. The choice is up to us.

Resources for Independent Living

Design Without Limits – a book from Simplicity Pattern Company on how to fill the special clothing needs of the disabled. Published by Drexel Design Press. Offers instructions on how to adjust home sewing patterns and adapt ready-to-wear clothing; also lists sources for supplies and special aids for various garment needs. Write: Simplicity's Design Without Limits, P.O. Box 2102, Niles, MI 49120-8102. $14.95.

Creative Cooking Cookbook for the Challenged – from Positive Approach, Inc., a nonprofit group serving the disabled and handicapped. For those wheelchair-bound or suffering from arthritis. Write: Positive Approach, Inc., 1600 Malone, Millville Airport, N.J. 08332. $10.00.

Independent Living Aids Catalog – for the blind, hearing impaired, arthritic, diabetic, handicapped. Write: Independent Living Aids, Inc., 27 East Mall, Plainview, N.Y. 11803 or call 1-800-537-2118.

Directory of Travel Agencies for the Disabled – lists more than 350 agencies in the U.S., Canada and world wide that specialize in arranging travel for people with disabilities. Write: The Disability Bookshop, P.O. Box 129, Vancouver, WA. 98666. $19.95 plus $2.00 shipping.

Access Travel: Airports – lists facilities and services for the handicapped at 519 airport terminals in 62 countries. Write: Dept. 584R, Consumer Information Center, Pueblo, Co. 81009.

The OPT Report – a travel newsletter from the non-profit "Organization For the Promotion of Access and Travel for the Handicapped." Annual membership fee of $15.00. Free list of cruise ships with wheelchair-accessible cabins and list of information on wheelchairs suitable for onboard. Write: OPT P.O. Box 15777, Tampa, FL 33684.

Fitness

Nancy's Special Workout for the Physically Challenged – (45 minutes, aerobic). $39.95, P.O. Box 2914, Southfield, MI 48037-2914, (313)682-5511.

Armchair Fitness – (three twenty-minute stretching and strengthening workouts.) $42.45 CC-M Productions, P.O. Box 15707 Dept. G., Chevy Chase, MD 20815-0707, (301)588-4095.

Keep Fit While You Sit – (33 minutes aerobic and upper-body strengtheners.) $29.50, Slabo Productions, 1057 S. Crescent Heights Blvd., Los Angeles, CA 90035, (213) 935-8624.

Sit and Be Fit – (45 minutes, strengthening, flexibility and aerobic segments.) $42.95, 10201 N. 58th Place, Scottsdale, AZ 85253, (602)998-8455.

Strength and Flexibility Exercises for All Types of Disabilities – (60 minutes) $29.50, National Handicapped Sports, 1145 19th St. N.W., Suite 717, Washington, D.C., 20036, (202) 652-7505.

Audiocassettes

Wheelchair Workout with Janet Reed – (30 minutes, stretching and strengthening exercise, plus manual.) $16.75, 12275 Greenleaf Ave., Potomac, MD 20854, (301)279-2994.

The Exercise Program – (60 minutes, toning and strengthening workout, plus manual.) $32.95, Demos Publications, 156 Fifth Ave., Ste 1018, New York, N.Y. 10010, (212)255-8768.

FINISHING WELL

". . . that I may finish my race with joy, and the ministry which I received from the Lord Jesus."

Acts 20:24

The contrast between finishing poorly and finishing well was expressed in a poem by Robertson McQuilkin, who wrote:

The darkness of a spirit
  grown mean and small, fruit shriveled on the vine,
  bitter to the taste of my companions,
  burden to be borne by the brave few who love me still.
No, Lord. Let the fruit grow lush and sweet,
  a joy to all who taste;
Spirit-sign of God at work–
  stronger, fuller, brighter at the end.
Lord, let me get home before dark.

Alexander Schindler says the art of living is "to know when to hold fast and when to let go."

For life is a paradox: it enjoins us to cling to its many gifts even while it ordains their eventual relinquishment. Surely we ought to hold fast to life, for it is wondrous, and full of a beauty that breaks through every pore of God's own earth.

We know that this is so, but all too often we recognize this truth only in our backward glance when we remember what was and then suddenly realize it is no more.

We remember a beauty that faded, a love that waned. But we remember with far greater pain that we did not see that beauty when it flowered, that we failed to respond to love when it was tendered.

Here then is the first pole of life's paradoxical demands on us: Never be too busy for the wonder and the awe of life. Be reverent before each dawning day. Embrace each hour. Seize each golden moment.

Hold fast to life . . . but not so fast that you cannot let go. This is the second side of life's coin, the opposite pole of its paradox: we must accept our losses, and then learn to let go.

This is not an easy lesson to learn, especially when we are young and think that the world is ours to command, that whatever we desire with the full force of our passionate being can, nay *will*, be ours. But then life moves along to confront us with realities, and slowly but surely this second truth dawns upon us.

At every stage of life we sustain losses – and grow in the process. We begin our independent lives only when we emerge from the womb and lose its protective shelter. We enter a progression of schools; then we leave our fathers and mothers and our childhood homes. We get married and have children and then have to let them go. We confront the death of our parents and our spouses. We face the gradual or not so gradual waning of our own strength. And ultimately, as the parable of the open and closed hand suggests, we must confront the inevitability of our own demise, losing ourselves as it were, all that we were or dreamed to be.

But why should we be reconciled to life's contradictory demands? Why fashion things of beauty when beauty is evanes-

cent? Why give our hearts in love when those we love will ultimately be torn from our grasp?

In order to resolve this paradox, we must seek a wider perspective, viewing our lives as through windows that open on
eternity. Once we do that, we realize that our deeds on earth
weave a timeless pattern.

Life is never just a being. It is a becoming, a relentless flow-
ing-on. Our parents live on through us, and we will live on
through our children. The institutions we build endure, and we
will endure through them. The beauty that we fashion cannot
be dimmed by death. Our flesh may perish, our hands will with-
er, but that which we create in beauty and goodness and truth
lives on for all time.[1]

NOT WHY, BUT WHAT?

When trouble or trying circumstances come our way, we
often ask, "Why did this happen to me?" It would be better if
we would ask, "What can I learn from this? What is God teach-
ing me?"

Ruth Paxson, missionary to China during the first part of this
century, told of a woman who boarded a train with her in Finland. The first thing Miss Paxson noticed was her radiant face.
But then she observed that the woman's right hand was miss-
ing, and in its place was a steel hook. As they talked, Miss
Paxson learned that she had been a missionary in India, had
contracted a lung disease, and had been sent home to die. So
she returned to her native Finland, bought a farm, and worked
vigorously. One day, while she was working on the threshing
machine, her right hand was cut off. Now, as the two talked on
board the train, she told Miss Paxson, "When my hand was cut
off, I immediately looked up to my Lord and said, 'Lord, what
do you want me to do now that my right hand is gone? What

work? I'm not asking why, but what?' " God used her to turn her farm into a home for elderly Christians, bringing blessing to many.[2]

BLESSINGS OF ILLNESS

We can be a blessing or a burden to others in our illness. There are also some blessings that can come to us through illness, if we will only look for them and ask the Lord to show them to us. Here are a few:

1) *We have an opportunity to be an inspiration to others.*

If it means pain and suffering, that doesn't sound like much of an honor, does it? But we need to ask ourselves, have we ever had a pastor, teacher, coach or friend who was an inspiration to us? We need to think of how much good that person's influence did in our lives. We can be that source of good for another. We *can* get through this, and by doing so, we can help someone else get through their trial.

2) *Illness or disability will force us to slow down and seek God's will more, possibly even for the first time.*

We all make such plans. I'm going to be . . . I'm going to do . . . I'm going to go . . . Illness can ruin the best laid plans in life, and then we have to stop and ask ourselves if the direction we've been heading in is really God's perfect plan for us. There is one, if we'll seek it out. It may not be the easiest one, but if it's God-designed, it will fit us like a glove. Illness will stop us in our tracks, and God may do this to turn us around in the opposite direction. Or He may be telling us to get off the tracks completely. Or maybe we've just been sitting on the tracks too long, doing nothing. People who sit on tracks get run over. That's not God's plan for us. When we slow down we can hear that still, small voice speak.

3) Illness will force us to grow emotionally.

Have we always been the kind who run from challenges; shirking responsibility, or refusing to accept reality? Perhaps the Lord is going to use this time to show us our shortcomings. Chronic illness isn't for "sissies." It's the Big Leagues – we have to go to bat, grit our teeth, and determine that we're going to win. And only *we* can make the choice to do this.

> Dear brothers, is your life full of difficulties and temptations? Then be happy, for when the way is rough, your patience has a chance to grow. So let it grow, and don't try to squirm out of your problems. For when your patience is finally in full bloom, then you will be ready for anything, strong in character, full and complete. (James 1:2-4, LB).

4) Illness will force us to closely examine our faith and give us the opportunity to grow spiritually.

Do we really believe that God is sovereign and in control? Or have we just given this concept lip service over the years, and now that we're in a jam, we're ready to pack up and go home? It was God's will for 11 of 12 disciples to die martyr's deaths. This was not an easy road. Today's Christianity often teaches us that everything should be easy and go "our way," but that is not what Scripture teaches. We must ask ourselves, "Has this happened to me without God's knowledge or consent?" and then be willing to face the truth of what He may be trying to do in our lives.

5) God can get glory through our illness or disability.

As Christians, we are always to be an example to others of

the Lord's mighty power within us. But illness gives us a special platform that we would never have had as healthy people. People can look at our lives and see just how well we're doing, and instantly make a judgment about the power of the Lord in our lives. That's a big responsibility, but it's also a big opportunity. We never know who's watching or when. It's when "The rubber hits the road" in life that people's true colors shine through. I have a friend from school who is not a Christian, and we drifted apart because she just couldn't understand "that Christianity thing." She chose to be friends with people who were less threatening to her comfort-zone in life. Recently, she became ill. And who was it she called? Not her non-Christian friends . . . they had nothing to offer her. It was me. "You seem so happy," she said, "How do you do it?"

What an opportunity to witness! And what a score for the Lord . . . because He was the source of my happiness, and the One who had brought me through.

And this is my prayer for you . . . that through God's grace and strength you will become an Overcomer, not merely "getting by," but being *used* . . . and that you can be for someone else, somewhere down the line, what you needed – a strong, faithful, loving, supportive, growing, productive Child of God who will take them by the hand, tell them, "I'm praying for you," (and then will *do it*) and will see to it that they know they are loved and cared about, through it all. Give someone the gift of listening, *really* listening to their rantings and ravings, their pain and fears and loss . . . this is the most basic, precious gift you can give, one that maybe only *you* can give now.

We really do need each other. . . .

. . . live in vital union with him. Let your roots go down deep into him and draw up nourishment from him. See that you go on growing in the Lord, and become strong and vigorous in the truth you were taught. Let your lives overflow with joy and thanksgiving for all he has done (Col. 2:6,7, LB).

1. Schindler, Alexander M., "Two Truths to Live By," *Speeches of the Day,* (August 15, 1987).
2. "Not Why, But What?" Paul R. Van Gorder Vol. 31, No. 6,7, Sept. 1986. Used by permission Radio Bible Class.

In Memorium
Judith Mary O'Brien
1937 — 1991

Lady warrior
Smiling friend
You might not have won, but your struggle was sublime.
If I ever thought I wasn't making it
I had only to look at you.

Did you really think that if you said "I hurt . . . I need,"
That no one would love you anymore?
You were a master at making us think you were invincible
And then like cold splintered glass you were gone.

But, wait! I want to cry
I didn't know . . . couldn't see
We all play the game, say the right words
You couldn't have meant it when you said you had given up.

But you did.
If only I had listened beyond the words
I wouldn't have to feel guilty
That I selfishly took your smile for granted.

Rest sweetly. You are missed.

C.M.

Perfect sincerity and transparency make a great part of beauty,
as in dewdrops, lakes and diamonds.

–Thoreau

Facts on Chronic Illness and Disability

Multiple Sclerosis

500,000 are believed to have MS or related diseases.

In a national survey, four out of ten patients left the work force or were dismissed from their jobs.

In 1976, the average MS patient lost 44% of his or her income to the disease.

Approximately 9,500 new cases are reported each year.

50% of the patients surveyed cannot get around by themselves.

Indications: bladder dysfunction, sexual dysfunction
              spasticity, overwhelming fatigue, tremors,
              loss of coordination, numbness, vision problems

(Information from the Information and Resource Library, the National Multiple Sclerosis Society.)

Systemic Lupus Erythematosus

50,000 new cases are diagnosed annually.

According to one study, the average time between the onset of Lupus symptoms and correct diagnosis is five years.

Doctors often refer patients to psychiatrists because the disease is so difficult to diagnose. The vague, episodic nature of Lupus increases the chances of the doctor telling the patient, "It's all in your head."

Indications: skin rashes, often spreading over the entire face; fatigue, depression, hair loss, kidney dysfunction

(Stein, H., et al., "Systematic Lupus Erythematosus – A Medical and Social Profile," *The Journal of Rheumatology, 13:3, 1986.*)

C.E.B.V. (Chronic Epstein-Barr Virus Syndrome, a.k.a. Chronic Fatigue Syndrome.)

4 million Americans have been diagnosed with this disease.

Although some patients function slightly below par, others are too sickly to do the simplest of chores.

Symptoms fluctuate in severity, not only from month to month, but also day to day, leaving the patient and family unable to get a firm grasp on the illness.

Indications: Likened to a never-ending flu, the symptoms include extreme fatigue, aching, memory loss, inability to concen-

trate,muscular weakness, nausea, diarrhea, severe pain in the joints, sore throats, fever and chills.
(Information from the National C.E.B.V. Syndrome Assoc., Inc. Portland, Or.)

Rheumatoid Arthritis

7 million people have Rheumatoid Arthritis

It is three times more common in women than in men

A degenerative connective-tissue disease, it disables and can cripple: a 40 year-old woman may not be able to lift a frying pan, because her wrist would snap in two.

(Information, the Contra Costra [Ca.] Times, 4 July, 1988

Asthma

12 million people suffer from Asthma.

It causes significant disability in some sufferers: 15% of all Californians who have Asthma are incapacitated by the disease at least two months of every year.

Head injuries

Every 15 seconds someone in the United States suffers a head injury, usually from a fall, assault, or car accident.

One out of two of those victims will become permanently disabled.

More than 2 million Americans annually suffer a head injury. Of those who survive, 70,000 to 90,000 will endure a lifetime of disability.

(Information, Department of Health and Human Services.)

Disabilities

Over 1,000 Americans are severely hurt in accidents every hour, with a yearly toll of about 350,000 victims.

One out of six adults between the ages of 18-64 are disabled due to accident or chronic illness.

(Information, National Safety Council.)

NOTE: This list is not meant to be inclusive, but a sampling of the millions of people who struggle with chronic illness and disability daily.

What if the doctor told you that you weren't going to die—but would never get well? This book is written by someone who has been there, someone who has lived the roller-coaster life of the chronically ill.

This book is to help those who are sick and disabled come to grips with the pain, misunderstanding, and seeming hopelessness of the situation. It is to help them gain a clearer understanding of the need to restructure their lives, restructure their faith, and come to accept the reality of a divine plan for illness in their lives.

Binding Up The Brokenhearted will comfort those who most need to be comforted and help to restore life's balance which can be lost in suffering.

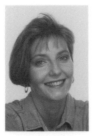

Cynthia L. Moench is a homemaker living in Antioch, Calif. with her husband, Jim. She owned and operated a floral business until nine years ago when she contracted Chronic Fatigue Syndrome and was no longer able to work. She has written articles for several periodicals and completed one novel.

COLLEGE PRESS PUBLISH
P.O. Box 1132, Joplin, Mi

ISBN: 0-89900-399